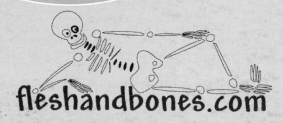

Respiratory Medicine

Commissioning Editor: Michael Parkinson
Project Development Manager: Jim Killgore
Project Manager: Frances Affleck
Designer: Sarah Russell
Page Layout: Archetype Graphic Communication, Peebles, Scotland

AN ILLUSTRATED COLOUR TEXT

Respiratory Medicine

Colin D. Selby DM FRCPE

Consultant Physician
Respiratory and Intensive Care Medicine
Queen Margaret Hospital
Dunfermline, UK

Illustrated by MTG

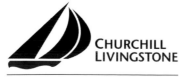

CHURCHILL
LIVINGSTONE

EDINBURGH   LONDON   NEW YORK   PHILADELPHIA   ST LOUIS   SYDNEY   TORONTO   2002

CHURCHILL LIVINGSTONE
An imprint of Elsevier Science Limited

First published 2002

ISBN 0443-05949-7

British Library Cataloguing in Publication Data
A catalogue record for this book is available from the British Library.

Library of Congress Cataloging in Publication Data
A catalog record for this book is available from the Library of Congress.

Note
Medical knowledge is constantly changing. As new information becomes available, changes in treatment, procedures, equipment and the use of drugs become necessary. The authors and the publishers have, as far as it is possible, taken care to ensure that the information given in this text is accurate and up-to-date. However, readers are strongly advised to confirm that the information, especially with regard to drug usage, complies with the latest legislation and standards of practice.

The
publisher's
policy is to use
**paper manufactured
from sustainable forests**

Printed in China by RCD Group Limited

PREFACE

This is but one in the series 'Illustrated Colour Text' developed by Churchill Livingstone. I have intended that it illustrates some of the visual appeal, breadth and challenges of respiratory medical practice. I have used a sequence from structure and function through clinical approaches to disease categories.

Images have been chosen to balance the text and relate to the clinical material. The presence of a number of radiographs reflects my view of the crucial inter-relationship between the practice of radiology and that of clinical respiratory medicine. Much of the thorax we see is via radiological images.

The case histories are a constant feature through this book's sections. I have intended that they add an additional clinical dimension, based as they are on real dilemmas. Their answers include tips and sometimes a little further material for thought.

They can be read with the section concerned or approached as a way of clinical revision.

This book should appeal to undergraduate medical students, clinical nurse specialists and primary care physicians. Postgraduate medical staff may appreciate some of the material; the case histories may be useful exam practice. It would sit comfortably on the bookshelf of medical wards. Though of European gestation it should appeal to an international audience.

Though any errors are mine, any comments or suggestions for change would be welcome.

Edinburgh
2002

Colin D Selby

ACKNOWLEDGEMENTS

An Illustrated Colour Text is dependent upon its illustrations. I consider myself lucky to have worked with, and am grateful for the technical expertise and advice of both Julie Close and Norman McMullan of the Medical Photography and Illustration Unit, Queen Margaret Hospital.

Colleagues raided their own image collections to fill particular gaps in mine. Drs Robin Smith (Fig. 3 p. 20), Katherine Jamieson (Fig. 1, p. 24), Ian Laurenson (Fig. 2 p. 25), Gemma Rebello (Fig. 2 p. 54) and Mr Bill Walker (Fig. 4 p. 67 and Fig. 1 p. 72) deserve appreciation.

Artists at Churchill Livingstone developed my sketches with true professionalism.

Past and present students, trainees and colleagues have allowed me to test explanations, arguments and diagrams.

Finally to Jackie, Fiona and Laura for their support during the gestation of this project.

CONTENTS

SPECIAL TOPICS   76

APPENDIX   80

CASE HISTORY COMMENTS   84

INDEX   87

THE CHALLENGES OF RESPIRATORY MEDICINE

WORLD-WIDE PERSPECTIVE

TOBACCO

The world is facing a global pandemic of tobacco-related mortality and morbidity. It is estimated that about a third of the global population aged over 14 are smokers; the majority (8×10^9) live in developing countries. Effects of tobacco control have been slight.

The development of mass production of cigarettes and matches in the early part of the 20th century represents a milestone in tobacco economics. With effective advertising, markets have been developed around the world where none existed before. Targeting the then largest population on earth, China, British American Tobacco (BAT) exploits in the first half of the 20th century were similar to the Western dissemination of opium into the same country a century earlier.

Nicotine, the addictive constituent of tobacco smoke, is readily absorbed across the alveolar–capillary barrier. It's pleasurable, with mainly central nervous system effects. It is as addictive as cocaine. Once started, the addiction ensures steady exposure over years to carcinogens and other damaging constituents. The lungs bear the brunt of the damage, as increased frequency of lung cancer and destruction as pulmonary emphysema.

Evidence for the health ill-effects of tobacco use started to accumulate from the early 1940s and have continued ever since. The most famous study has perhaps been the Doll and Hills longitudinal survey of British doctors over 40 years (1951–1991). Death from all causes in middle-aged smoking males was three times that of non-smokers. Other studies have added to the evidence not just of an excess mortality in smokers but of a dose response with increasing risk with increasing exposure as 'pack years'. The greatest risk is in those who start smoking regularly in their teenage years. To stop smoking is beneficial. The risk of malignancy falls with the passage of time to that of having never smoked after 10–15 years. The rate of decline in lung function at least lessens towards the age-related decline in function of non-smokers. Of immense concern is the knowledge that 50% of regularly smoking teenagers will be killed by their habit, and that 1 in 4 of 15-year-olds in the UK are already regular smokers.

The current issues relating to tobacco control are as much social and economic as medical, but they cannot be ignored by healthcare workers. Over 40 years from the first publication of its risk to health, tobacco is the leading preventable cause of death in developed countries and is almost that in the developing world. The trans-national tobacco corporations have increased their attentions to the developing countries, in part to replace the users lost in the developed countries through quitting and death. Death rates will therefore continue to rise well into the 21st century. The North American Tobacco company achieved $45 billion sales at a time when the pure medical costs of smoking-related illness cost the US $50 billion without counting the social and non-medical economic costs of illness and premature death. Of equal concern is that in 1993 the European Union spent 1.2 million ECU in the European fight against cancer via 'Europe against Cancer'. In the same financial year the subsidy for tobacco crops in Mediterranean EU countries was two orders of magnitude greater.

Strategies to limit the harm from tobacco have been various. They include aggressive taxation, banning smoking in the workplace and public areas, advertising bans and regulation as a drug. Increasingly stringent legal actions are proving effective in North America and are being initiated in the UK and Europe. Populations of many developing countries have no hope of such control measures.

TUBERCULOSIS (Tb)

The World Health Organization has described the current resurgence in tuberculosis infection as a world epidemic: 'the greatest public health hazard since the bubonic plague' (Fig. 1). In 1990, 2.9 million people died from this infection. Co-infection with HIV infection is lethal. Immunosuppression by HIV infection accelerates the progression of tuberculosis infection to clinical disease. Tb as an AIDS-defining illness promotes HIV infection to AIDS. Tuberculosis probably accelerates the decline in immunity due to HIV. The economically active adult population of sub-Saharan Africa is being decimated by this twinning, leaving the elderly and orphans unsupported. South East Asia, with Tb already endemic, is about to experience these consequences following the arrival there of HIV.

Multiply drug-resistant Tb (MDR-Tb) is a different but related issue where the infecting organism is resistant to at least two of the standard first-line antibiotics. Treatment is thus more difficult, involving the use of more toxic drugs. This is a major public health concern in Asia and in the city of New York where there have been deaths of healthcare workers due to MDR-Tb.

Treating tuberculosis is one of the most cost-effective healthcare interventions studied. As much of the disease is currently in developing countries, the global inequalities of wealth

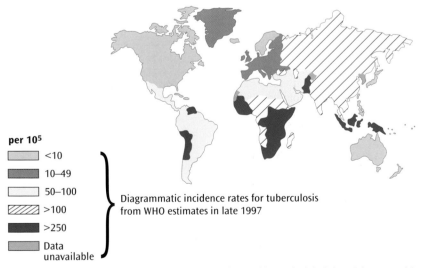

per 10^5

- <10
- 10–49
- 50–100
- >100
- >250
- Data unavailable

Diagrammatic incidence rates for tuberculosis from WHO estimates in late 1997

Fig. 1 **The global epidemic of tuberculosis.** In much of Africa and increasingly in Asia and the states of the former Soviet Union, co-infection with HIV is common. (Reproduced with permission from JAMA 1999; 282: p 683; copyrighted 1999, American Medical Association.)

and social infrastructure will need addressing for effective world-wide control. For the cost of one modern warplane a successful world-wide eradication programme could be funded!

OTHER INFECTIONS

Infections due to pneumococci are an important cause of world-wide mortality. The first clinical appearance of pneumococci resistant to penicillin (it is usually exquisitely susceptible) was in Australia in 1967. Subsequent spread in New Guinea by the late 1970s and into countries as diverse as Spain and South Africa is another reminder that we must not be therapeutically complacent with infections. Childhood respiratory infections are still a leading cause of mortality in the developing world.

AIR QUALITY

The thick 'pea soup' smogs of the 1950s have been banished from developed countries, but there is now increasing concern and evidence for the health ill-effects of air pollutants generated by industry and transportation and acted upon by UV sunlight to cause photochemical smogs. These pollutants include the oxides of nitrogen, benzene, ozone and respirable airborne carbonaceous particles (PM_{10}). Evidence has been accumulating that the combined effects of these pollutants exacerbate pre-existing lung diseases. It is proving more difficult to confirm or refute the concern that such pollutants may trigger de novo conditions such as asthma.

UK PERSPECTIVE

Morbidity

Roughly 1 in 6 of all general practice consultations in the United Kingdom are respiratory in nature, with at least 10% of primary care drug expenditure being on respiratory medication. Respiratory disease is now the most common reason for attending a general practitioner in the UK. A third of UK certified sickness incapacity is due to respiratory complaints, each with additional but immeasurable social costs (Table 1).

Table 1 **Respiratory disease in the UK: statistics**

- 33% of female sickness incapacity
- 10% of primary care drug prescriptions
- 30% of primary care consultations–the most common reason for attending
- Second only to skin disorders in occupationally-related disease
- 16% of UK adult mortality

Mortality

Respiratory disease contributes in excess of 10% of 'all cause' UK mortality. There is a steady increase with age rising above 30 years, amounting to nearly 20% in over 65-year-olds. In this age group, infections, obstructive airway diseases and cancer predominate.

Asthma

Delivering quality care and ensuring cost-effectiveness in asthma treatment remain challenges in finance-limited healthcare systems and topics of current debate.

Lung cancer

Lung cancer is increasing and has become the most common cause of cancer death in males in the UK. Mechanisms of care delivery to such patients continue to be explored. Cigarette smoking is the cause in the majority of these patients. In contrast to the costs of caring for patients with lung cancer or other tobacco-related

diseases, proportionately little is spent on effective primary prevention. Preventing teenagers starting the habit is the most cost-effective approach. An aggressive pricing policy, effective advertising restrictions and effective support for people wishing to give up the habit cannot be underestimated (Fig. 2).

THE FUTURE

Advances in our understanding of disease processes through techniques in molecular biology are allowing novel therapies to be developed and tested. Trials of gene replacement therapy in cystic fibrosis and protein replacement therapy for α_1-proteinase inhibitor (α_1Pi) deficiency are underway. The challenges of tobacco control, maximising currently available and clinically effective therapy coupled with the continued development of novel therapies will continue to challenge medicine and respiratory medicine in particular well into this millennium.

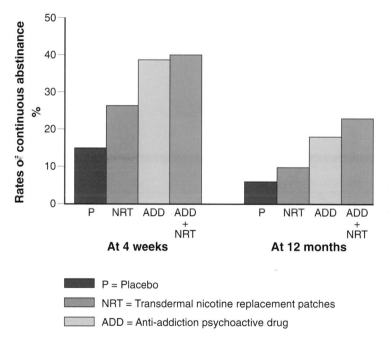

P = Placebo
NRT = Transdermal nicotine replacement patches
ADD = Anti-addiction psychoactive drug

Fig. 2 **Examples of rates of continuous quitting from tobacco smoking with a range of 9-week courses of anti-smoking therapies.** The benefit of not ever smoking can be easily seen.

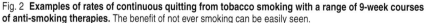

The challenges of respiratory medicine

- Smoking is the greatest preventable cause of death world-wide. Its risks are greatest in those who start young and continue. To stop smoking works.
- Smoking cessation programmes the world over are not receiving the financial support they deserve.
- Tuberculosis remains an important global threat to health.
- Issues of clinical delivery of care and cost-effectiveness will increasingly require addressing.

ANATOMY AND VENTILATION

EMBRYOLOGY AND GROSS ANATOMY

The lungs with their branching airways and alveoli develop from buds arising off the foregut early in embryological development. Some of these branches abort early to produce blind-ending, bronchial pits. Other branchings may produce additional or accessory pulmonary lobules or even lobes. An inadequately developed lung segment may be sequestered within otherwise normal lung tissue as a 'sequestration'. These are usually linked to the bronchial tree but have an anomalous blood supply. If infection enters via the bronchial connection it will never be eradicated and careful surgical resection will have to be considered.

In utero, the lungs develop in a fluid medium. Surfactant is crucially required when respiration commences to reduce alveolar closure. It is secreted late in uterine development. Infants born prematurely are at risk of developing respiratory distress as a result of stiff, uninflatable lungs. Synthetic preparations of surfactant coupled with improvements in neonatal intensive care have increased chances of survival for these infants.

The lungs continue to develop well into childhood. Early postnatal exposure to infections and inhaled irritants such as tobacco smoke adversely affect lung maturation. Thus the physiological peak reached in the early 20s is reduced and from which the age-related decline occurs with any acceleration by additional lung injury.

RESPIRATION

This is the process of drawing ambient atmosphere into the lungs and delivering oxygen to aerobically metabolising (oxygen-utilising) cells. Waste carbon dioxide is then removed as part of the process. Respiration can be considered as:

- ventilation, with mass movement of air
- gas exchange, oxygen uptake, by diffusion
- oxygen transportation and delivery to tissues
- carbon dioxide removal.

VENTILATION

Air is drawn through the upper respiratory tract and along conducting airways to replenish the alveolar gas volume.

The nose

The nose warms and humidifies the inspired air as well as trapping debris particles. If viruses or pollen are trapped a local immune response may be triggered. The inspired air is warmed by being drawn over richly vascularised turbinates that act as baffles. Humidification is achieved from a mucosa that is rich in secretory cells and mucus glands that produce a surface layer of mucus. This epithelium is lined with cilia that move the surface layer of mucus and deposited debris in a conveyor belt-like manner back towards the nasopharynx (Fig. 1).

The larynx

The epiglottis is an important shield over the vocal cords and the trachea (Fig. 2). During swallowing, boluses of food and liquid are deflected around the trachea inlet and down into the oesophagus. In adults, breathing and swallowing are under separate and voluntary control. By contrast in a suckling neonate, nasal breathing and swallowing occur simultaneously.

The vocal cords move gently during ventilation. They are under voluntary control during phonation when ventilation is co-ordinated with speech. Their control is involuntary during the cough reflex. Abnormalities of the cord surface or of their movement alter the character of the voice. Innervation is by the recurrent laryngeal nerves. While the right remains outside the thorax, the left loops down adjacent to the mediastinum to below the aortic arch before ascending to the larynx. Pathological disease, especially malignancy, there will damage the nerve and paralyse the left vocal cord.

A cough is initiated by irritation of nociceptive nerve endings within the mucosa of the major conducting airways. The vocal cords are closed tightly together. Active contraction of the expiratory muscles then rapidly increases pressure within the thorax. When the cords fly open, air is rapidly and audibly expelled together with any irritating particulate matter. Paralysis of either cord prevents the effective increase in intrathoracic pressure necessary for the explosive release of the cough itself. The cough is ineffective and sounds bovine.

AIR MOVEMENT

Respiratory muscle pump

Inspiration. Mass movement of air into the lungs is achieved by active inspiration. The respiratory muscle pump comprises the diaphragm, intercostal muscles and shoulder girdle, acting upon the skeletal thorax. Effective contraction of these muscle groups expands the thoracic cavity and the lungs are drawn out from their resting volume by surface tension at the pleural surfaces (Fig. 3). This generates a negative pressure within the thorax and a potential negative pressure at the pleurae. Air is drawn along the conducting airways by this pressure gradient from atmosphere to thorax. In quiet respiration, the volume of air moved is around 7 ml.kg^{-1} with pressure change of a few cm H$_2$O. This is tidal breathing.

Expiration is predominantly passive. The inspiratory muscles relax and the elasticity of the inflated lung recoils to a smaller volume. The maximum volume inspired from a full expiration is termed vital capacity. Minute ventilation at rest, the

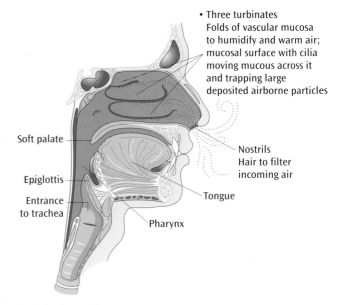

• Three turbinates
Folds of vascular mucosa to humidify and warm air; mucosal surface with cilia moving mucous across it and trapping large deposited airborne particles

Nostrils
Hair to filter incoming air

Soft palate

Epiglottis

Entrance to trachea

Tongue

Pharynx

Fig. 1 **Anatomy of the nose.**

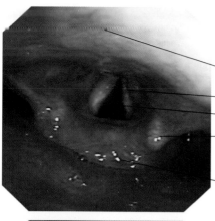

View of larynx looking toward vocal cords and entrance to trachea

— Posterior surface of epiglottis

— Right vocal cord

— To trachea

— Arytenoid cartilage (articulated for cord movement)

— Bubbles at entrance to oesophagus

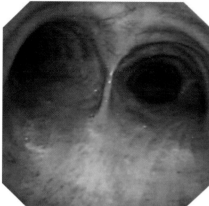

Carina
Birfurcation at lower end of trachea to left main and right main bronchi (dividing into upper and intermediate bronchi). 'Horseshoes' of supporting cartilage in tracheal wall can be seen. The posterior floor is unsupported. Its muscles bow in on coughing and to allow passage of food boluses in oesophagus

Lower lobe bronchi supporting bronchopulmonary segments
Sharp divisions, branching structure and hoops of cartilage as supports can all be seen clearly

Fig. 2 **Larynx and conducting airways.**

tively by decreased neuromuscular function with decreased respiratory drive or neuromuscular incompetence.

A respiratory control centre in the base of the brain maintains cyclical breathing. It receives its information from receptors sensitive to stretch and movement in the respiratory muscles and within the lungs. The chemistry of the blood and surrounding cerebrospinal fluid is also a factor that affects the rate and depth of ventilation. There is also the ability for conscious control during activities such as speech and exercise. Output to the main respiratory muscles is via the phrenic nerve and intercostal nerves to the diaphragm and intercostal muscles respectively. The phrenic nerve originates from the lower cervical cord and is at risk from neck injuries.

Muscle function may be depressed by such factors as:

- drugs
- electrolyte disturbances especially potassium, magnesium, phosphate or acidosis
- neuromuscular disease.

Respiratory muscle function can be measured. The ability of the diaphragm to displace the abdominal contents without the assistance of gravity as a postural vital capacity can be compared to a vital capacity effort made vertically. Alternatively, the measurement is taken of the most negative pressure generated within the thorax by a short, sharp, inspiratory attempt such as a sniff.

Chronic inflammation of the rib–spinal joints may lead to bone union that fixes the thoracic cage. Subsequent respiratory movement is only by the diaphragm.

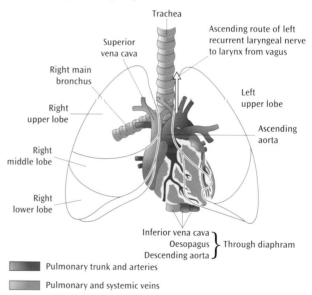

Fig. 3 **Anatomy of the thorax.**

product of breath volume and breath frequency, is around 5 l per minute.

Effective respiration requires intact nerve and muscle function, patent airways and a thoracic shape that allows effective muscle action. Respiratory failure arises either because of increased load upon the pump by airway narrowing or lung stiffening, or alterna-

---

Case history 1

A 68-year-old male smoker is admitted with a few months of increasing breathlessness and a few days of hoarseness. An urgent ear, nose and throat surgical review by indirect laryngoscopy confirms a left vocal cord palsy. The chest radiograph demonstrates a mass adjacent to the left hilum.
Why?

Anatomy and ventilation

- Lung growth and development continues well into teenage years. Exposure to severe infections or inhaled irritants may adversely affect lung maturation.
- Vocal cord surface changes or abnormalities of their movement will affect an individual's voice.
- Effective respiration requires intact nerve and muscle function, patent airways and a thoracic shape that allows effective muscle action.
- Respiratory muscle function can be measured by means of either a postural vital capacity or the negative pressure exerted upon a maximal sniff manoeuvre.

AIRFLOW AND DELIVERY

CONDUCTING AIRWAYS

Gas moves forwards and backwards along airways that start as the trachea and progressively branch into smaller airways to bronchioles. The large airways provide a further opportunity after the nose for warming and humidification. They are supported against expiratory collapse by cartilage within their walls. They are richly innervated with plentiful mucous glands and epithelial goblet cells. Smooth muscle surrounds these airways.

Debris, dust and microbes may land upon the walls, where they are caught up in a flow of mucus driven by the cilia of the surface cells. This 'mucociliary escalator' moves up towards the larynx where the mucous mix may be coughed up or swallowed. Many of the inhaled particles impinge upon and around the sites of branching of the airways. Microbes may evade this defence by penetrating the mucous barrier and paralyse the 'escalator'.

Disease processes in the large airways have been more readily understood, particularly with the use of flexible bronchoscopy that allows access to these sites. Recently there has been increasing realisation of the importance of the small distal airways in healthy resistance to flow and in airway diseases.

Measurement of airflow

Airflow can be measured routinely in clinical practice. **Spirometry** allows volume–time data collection and analysis on an expiratory forced vital capacity manoeuvre (Fig. 1). Flow data collected during inspiration and expiration can also be displayed as a flow–volume 'loop' (Fig. 2).

An individual's age, sex and height with a little allowance for ethnic origin determine 'normal' values for volumes and flows. All such reference values have a standard deviation that should be used to determine a reference range for the measured result.

Physiologically, the limitation of airflow is the commonest respiratory abnormality and is caused by airway obstruction or narrowing. Bronchial narrowing may be generalised or focal. Sputum plugs, tumour or an inhaled foreign body may cause localised obstruction. Generalised narrowing is usually caused by one of the two commonest respiratory disease processes: asthma or chronic obstructive pulmonary disease (COPD).

Airway obstruction

Mucosal oedema, airway smooth muscle contraction, enlargement of vascular spaces within the mucosa with epithelial shedding and increased mucus secretion will cause airway obstruction. Alternatively, destruction and loss of airway supports will also cause obstruction and airway collapse. Airway calibre is slightly less on expiration. Any further narrowing will increase the tendency for airway collapse. Hence, in the early stages airflow is limited but expired gas volumes are preserved. With increasing obstruction, gas trapping occurs behind narrow bronchi that close on expiration, reducing exhaled gas volumes to below predicted levels (Fig. 3). Direct measurement of airway resistance is possible but rarely fruitful in ordinary clinical practice.

Airway obstruction, collapse and subsequent distal gas trapping over time lead to a permanently overinflated thorax. The intercostal respiratory muscles then become overstretched and the diaphragm flattened. This forces them both to operate at mechanical disadvantages and create the potential for chronic ventilatory insufficiency.

Measurement of ventilated lung volume

Ventilated lung volume is usually measured by the dilution of a non-respirable, inert, tracer gas such as helium. The subject breathes in a closed system containing a known concentration of helium. After sufficient time for equilibration, the new steady state concentration of helium is measured. The resulting dilution corresponds to residual lung volume. Although the dilution of helium is the most utilised means, it can only measure the volume of ventilated lung. Lung units that are ventilated either poorly or not at all cannot contribute to the dilution of helium. The total intrathoracic gas volume can be measured by plethysmography in a 'body box'. This technique is not widely available and is technically demanding.

GAS DELIVERY

In the more distal parts of the lung, the small airways and into the alveoli, the mass movement of air gives way to diffusion. This process of diffusion is rarely limiting except occasionally in emphysema when the damaged airspaces become so large that the distance over which diffusion has to occur is so great that it contributes to hypoxia.

The functional part of the lungs is the alveolus. Here alveolar gas is replenished with each inspiration. It is separated from pulmonary capillary blood by the thinnest of possible layers: an alveolar epithelial cell, an endothelial cell and a minimal basement membrane. This alveolar–capillary barrier is maintained by an elastin-rich, lattice support slung between adjacent airways.

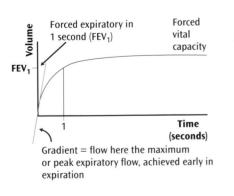

Fig. 1 **Spirometry.** Volume measured directly to time; in this case a normal forced expiration.

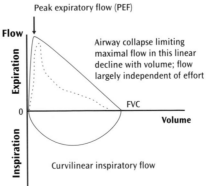

Fig. 2 **Flow–volume loops.** These illustrate flow at expired or inspired volume for normal and in airway obstruction.

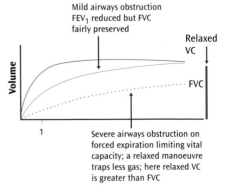

Fig. 3 **Airway obstruction.**

Virtually the entire cardiac output passes through this capillary bed. At rest in a healthy adult it is around 5 l per minute and the transit time of blood along a capillary segment is more than enough for the liberation of waste carbon dioxide. However, the uptake of oxygen is slower. Occasionally, in disease and during vigorous exercise, the oxygen requirements may exceed even this capability for uptake.

Reduced oxygen uptake in disease is more often the result of mismatching ventilation with blood delivery. In health, the 5 l of overall ventilation is fairly uniformly distributed throughout the lungs. The approximately equivalent blood flow delivered to both lungs at rest is distributed in favour of the bases as a result of gravity affecting the low-pressure, pulmonary circulation. This produces a slight ventilation-to-perfusion mismatch. More important mismatches occur in disease, creating two extreme possibilities (Fig. 4).

1 Areas of lung may be ventilated but not perfused: 'dead space'. This occurs physiologically in the large conducting airways. If it occurs substantially in the alveoli, perhaps as a result of pulmonary vascular bed occlusion, ventilation is wasted.
2 Perfusion of lung regions that are not ventilated: effectively, a right-to-left shunt with deoxygenated blood conducted directly into the systemic circulation. The oxygen–haemoglobin dissociation curve means that overventilation of other perfused lung regions cannot compensate for this mismatch.

Measurement of the matching of ventilation and perfusion

A measure of the overall matching of ventilation to perfusion is the carbon monoxide (CO) transfer test. This was initially devised to measure the perceived barrier to diffusion across the alveolar–capillary membrane. It is now seen as reflecting the matching of perfusion and ventilation. The subject inhales a gas mixture that includes a trace of carbon monoxide together with helium and oxygen. The latter allows determination of alveolar volume by gas dilution. The whole lung uptake of carbon monoxide is usually measured during a single breath. The difference in CO inhaled to that at the timed exhalation allows CO transfer expressed per minute and corrected for the gas gradient (T_{Lco}). The available haemoglobin and the alveolar volume for transfer are the major factors in the uptake of CO, the latter allowing gas transfer per unit of ventilated lung (K_{co}).

Restrictive respiratory disease

The other main group of respiratory disease is termed restrictive. This is a much more varied group and patient numbers are much smaller. Characteristically, loss of lung parenchyma occurs by destruction, fibrosis or infiltration. Airflow is usually preserved in proportion to the reduced lung volume. Volume is lost affecting vital capacity, total lung capacity and residual volume. The pathology that alters local ventilation and perfusion relationships usually leads to steadily deteriorating gas exchange, especially oxygenation (Fig. 5).

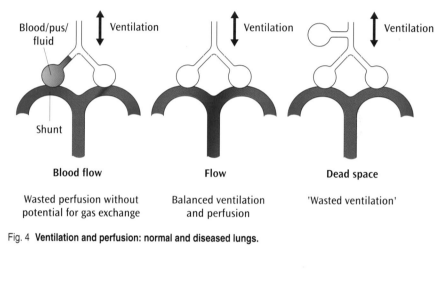

Fig. 4 **Ventilation and perfusion: normal and diseased lungs.**

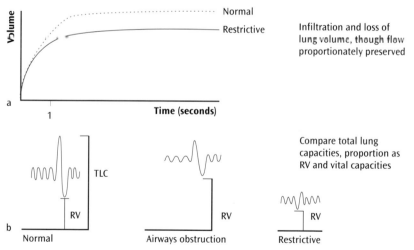

Fig. 5 **Infiltration and loss of lung volume, though flow proportionately preserved. (a)** Spirometry; **(b)** lung volumes.

Case history 2

A heavy smoker presents to clinic with progressive breathlessness over a decade. He is hypoxaemic at rest but spirometry is normal. Although his chest radiograph is unremarkable, imaging of his lung parenchyma by thin section CT scanning demonstrates widespread emphysema.
What is the explanation?

Airflow and delivery

- Pathophysiologically, airflow limitation is the commonest respiratory disturbance. It can be readily detected by means of spirometry.
- Gas exchange changes from mass movement of gas to diffusion the further down the branching airway tree to the alveoli one is.

GAS EXCHANGE

OXYGEN UPTAKE AND DELIVERY

The partial pressure of oxygen falls steadily at various sites along the 'route' from atmosphere to oxygen-metabolising, subcellular organelle. This pressure gradient can be considered as the head of pressure that drives oxygen movement. Deficiencies at any level may impact disastrously on the final step of oxygen availability for intracellular energy generation (Fig. 1).

Oxygen is taken across the alveolar–capillary membrane into passing erythrocytes. Here it is bound to haemoglobin, fitting within a conformational change of the molecule. Each haemoglobin molecule binds up to four oxygen molecules. The binding of each subsequent molecule eases the binding of the next. This is responsible for the sigmoid shape of the oxygen–haemoglobin dissociation curves that relate ambient partial pressure of oxygen to haemoglobin saturation. A little oxygen is transported directly dissolved within plasma.

Pulse oximetry

The saturation of pulsatile, systemic, arterial blood is now readily and non-invasively measurable in real time by transcutaneous or 'pulse' oximeters. These are exceedingly useful in clinical practice for measuring 'in real time' the adequacy of an individual's oxygenation. Modern sensors exhibit reasonable accuracy of ±3%, which can be readily checked on your own finger before measuring a patient.

However they require warm, well-perfused peripheries or mucous membranes across which to detect a pulsatile signal and measure reliably. Saturated oxyhaemoglobin is detected by its light transmission characteristics at a small number of specific wavelengths and quantified in relation to that of unsaturated haemoglobin. The pulsatile element of the total signal reflects that from arterial blood. The detectors can be confused by signals across abnormal haemoglobins. Carboxyhaemoglobin following carbon monoxide poisoning gives unreliable readings and methaemoglobin a characteristically consistent value of 85%.

Three clinically useful points are considered in Figure 2. It illustrates the nature of a sigmoid relationship and the importance of the 'knee' of the curve below which oxygen saturation (and hence content) fall precipitously in relation to

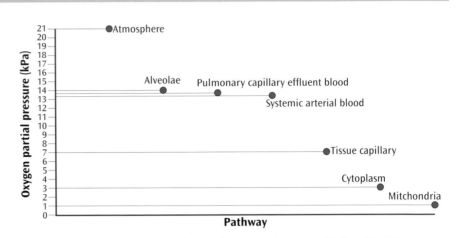

Fig. 1 **The gradient of partial pressure of oxygen from atmosphere to aerobically metabolising mitochondria.**

partial pressure. The alarm setting of most pulse oximeters defaults to 90–92% for that reason.

Saturation and delivery

The oxygen content of blood is clearly the sum of the oxygen bound to haemoglobin, reflected by its saturation and the remainder free within the plasma. The delivery of oxygen to tissues and organs is dependent upon both this oxygen content and the local flow of blood. All must be considered in terms of oxygen delivery. Maximising oxygen saturation is important but is of limited value if a patient's haemoglobin concentration is 25% of what it should be and cardiac output is failing.

CARBON DIOXIDE REMOVAL

Waste carbon dioxide is transported predominantly as bicarbonate ion in plasma. Carbonic acid is generated from the carbon dioxide in the vascular bed of metabolising tissues by the enzyme carbonic anhydrase. This also speeds the dissociation on to bicarbonate whence it is transported to the lungs. In the pulmonary capillaries, the carbonic anhydrase enzyme encourages the reversal of bicarbonate ion to carbon dioxide gas. Adequate ventilation washes out alveolar carbon dioxide to maintain a concentration gradient for diffusion. The arterial partial pressure of carbon dioxide is an indicator of ventilation and may be manipulated to alter the level of its associated acid (Fig. 3).

ACID–BASE BALANCE

Acute overventilation will blow off carbon dioxide and hence lower the level of carbonic acid. The resulting tendency to

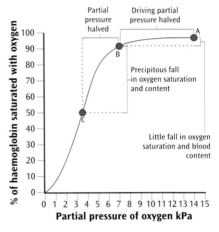

Fig. 2 **Relationship for oxygen between normal haemoglobin saturation and partial pressure.** Saturation is proportional to carriage and the product of that and blood flow relates to oxygen delivery. Ambient temperature and acidosis and type of haemoglobin alter the position of the curve slightly.

alkalosis is a useful response to a metabolic acidosis, attempting to minimise the acid–base disturbance. Such a response is rapid in onset, driven by the chemoreceptors inputting to the respiratory centre. However, it is usually incomplete, as the ability to compensate by overventilating is limited.

Acute underventilation results in carbon dioxide retention and an acute respiratory acidosis. Carbon dioxide excess behaves as a narcotic and as a vasodilator. However, it is the acidosis with any associated hypoxaemia that is more immediately life-threatening. Common causes are sedative drug excess, opiate analgesia or primary brain injury or inflammation. The problems of adequate oxygenation and of ventilation require addressing and both may be supported by mechanical ventilation.

Chronic respiratory insufficiency developing over months to years occurs typically in COPD. The slow deterioration allows compensatory mechanisms to develop that minimise any acid–base disturbance. The kidneys reclaim bicarbonate ion to neutralise the excess acid. This occurs slowly but the compensation is complete.

THE RESPIRATORY RESPONSE TO EXERCISE

The respiratory system responds to exercise by increasing oxygen uptake and delivery to active muscles and removes carbon dioxide with ease. Minute ventilation during heavy exercise can easily increase 10–20 fold (Fig. 4). This is achieved by a complex series of stimuli that include conscious elements, those from muscle and joints and those that are sensitive to changes in blood chemistry. Voluntarily, ventilation can be increased by an even greater extent. Blood therefore leaves the lungs fully saturated with oxygen even at maximal exertion, except in highly trained athletes when blood flow through the lungs may be so fast as to be unable to fully saturate it. Thus, in normal, healthy individuals, there is never any respiratory limitation to exercise. Hence, any arterial desaturation occurring on exercise indicates significant respiratory disease.

In health, it is the cardiovascular response that limits exercise. Cardiac output may increase by four to five times and respiring muscles extract a greater proportion of the oxygen delivered. However, with increasing workload, the inadequacy of oxygen delivery results in anaerobic metabolism. This releases lactic acid that can be detected in peripheral blood. The associated acidosis is buffered by bicarbonate to produce additional carbon dioxide that requires increased ventilation for its removal. This step increase in ventila-

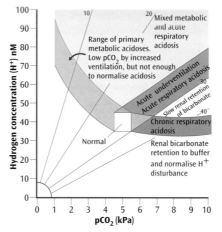

Fig. 3 **Primary acid–base and ventilation disorders and their secondary responses (after Flenley 1971).** Such a chart aids the clinical interpretation of real clinical values measured on arterial blood gas samples.

tion can be detected, is normal and is termed the 'anaerobic threshold'. It reflects inadequate perfusion.

In disease, exercise limitation occurs earlier; stiff lungs and airway obstruction increase the work of breathing. All three contribute to a patient's sensation of breathlessness. Hypoxia and hypercarbia also contribute to the sensation. This perception of breathlessness varies between individuals and the relationship between each of these factors is complex but unclear.

Regular exercise produces a number of health benefits. Physiologically, exercising muscles increases capillary density, in turn improving oxygen delivery and lactate threshold. The cardiovascular response is improved with better cardiac output and flows at lower heart rates with a better blood lipid profile. There are also beneficial responses that are less easy to quantify such as improved endurance and subjective well-being.

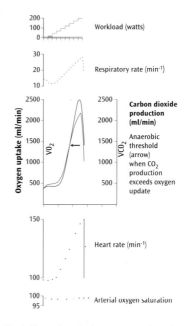

Fig. 4 **Normal respiratory response to submaximal workload.**

CARBON MONOXIDE POISONING

This inert, highly toxic gas is released during incomplete combustion. Poorly ventilated gas appliances or house fires are the commonest culprits. The gas binds avidly to haemoglobin preventing the carriage of oxygen. The clinical effects range from inconsequential reduction in the oxygen carrying capacity of the blood to severe coronary and cerebral hypoxia. Minor cerebral confusion, headaches through to coma from cerebral oedema are all possible. As pulse oximetry readings will be misleading, the carboxyhaemoglobin must be measured directly and therefore requires appreciation of CO poisoning as a possibility. Treatment requires high flow oxygen and possibly hyperbaric oxygen in severe cases. Chronic neuropsychiatric sequelae may result from severe poisoning.

Case history 3

A previously well, non-smoking middle-aged man presents to A&E. He is blue and this is confirmed when a pulse oximetry reading of 85% is obtained. He readily admits to having taken a drug overdose. He is completely orientated and his conversation and behaviours are appropriate.

What has happened?

Gas exchange

- Pulse oximetry is a readily portable and available means of measuring oxygen saturation. However, it can be fooled by abnormal haemoglobin whose presence is not suspected.
- The rapid respiratory response to a metabolic acidosis is prompt overventilation. This produces a partially compensating alkalosis.
- The metabolic response to a respiratory acidosis is renal retention of bicarbonate that is slow but corrects completely.
- The cardiovascular response, not the respiratory response, limits exercise capability in health.
- Carbon monoxide poisoning is an under-recognised cause of neuropsychiatric symptoms and is identified by specifically measuring carboxyhaemoglobin levels.

DEFENCE AND DISORDERED DEFENCE

A range of physical, chemical and cellular mechanisms are in place to protect the airways and parenchyma from injury consequent on inhaled particles including microbes (Fig. 1).

THE NOSE

This organ is the first line of protection (page 4). The effects of defective cilia function or abnormally tenacious mucus illustrate the importance of an effective 'mucociliary escalator,' even in the nose.

Dysmotile cilia syndromes

Cilia line the rhino–sino–pulmonary tree and the male vas deferens as well as being responsible for the orientation of the blastocyst early in embryological development. Defective function thus results in chronic sinusitis, bronchiectasis, male infertility and an evens chance of situs inversus.

Cilia beating and moving viscous mucus which is rich in bacterio-toxic proteins and enzymes, including lysozyme and anti-proteases

Intra-epithelial lymphocyte producing immunoglobulin

Oropharynx to main bronchi
- cough
- cilia and mucus
- lymph nodes behind airway branchings

Airways branching, resultant airflow turbulence and debris impaction

Alveoli
- immunoglobulin A
- alveolar macrophage
- T-lymphocytes
- Neutrophils in alveolar capillaries

Fig. 1 **Host defence mechanisms.**

Kartagener described the archetypal defect with loss of the dynein subunits involved in microfilament interaction for cilia movement. Subsequently, other de-fects in motility arising from abnormalities in microstructure or energy generation have been described.

Abnormally tenacious mucus is much rarer a problem but can cause a similar clinical picture. Detection of either dysmotile cilia or abnormal mucus is by the saccharin test. Having ensured that the individual is genetically able to taste saccharin, a tiny fragment is placed under direct vision upon one inferior turbinate. The time taken for the individual to taste

the sweetness is recorded as a result of the saccharin molecules being carried into the nasopharynx. A normal individual will be able to taste it within 30 minutes.

As well as inherited defects, pathogenic microbes and pollutants inhibit cilial function. *Pseudomonas* release chemicals that are particularly effective at paralysing ciliary action. Chronic sinopulmonary disease then occurs with chronic carriage and an inability to effectively eradicate the organism. Other respiratory pathogenic microbes including *Staphylococcus* and *Haemophilus* also interfere with ciliary action.

Flow and particulate dropout

The distance into the lungs travelled by inhaled particles relates to their effective aerodynamic size. The smaller the particle, the further into the lungs it will travel but also the more likely it is to be exhaled. At airway branchings, flow turbulence allows a particle to drop out and land upon the mucosa. Microbes, the fine particulate pollutants from diesel engine combustion known as PM_{10}'s and needle-like amphibole asbestos fibres all penetrate far into the small airways and alveoli.

NON-SPECIFIC ALVEOLAR DEFENCE

The major cell here is the roaming alveolar macrophage, derived from the circulating peripheral blood monocyte. These macrophages are able to engulf particles and kill intracellularly most ingested microbes. If the numbers of inhaled microbes are overwhelming, they are able to trigger an inflammatory response that includes recruitment of additional cells and a

heightened ability of the macrophages themselves to kill microbes.

Inflammation

An inflammatory response stimulates a broad cascade of responses from cells and chemicals. Although most inflammatory responses are directed against foreign material, occasionally host tissues at the site of inflammation or distant from it may be damaged as 'bystander' lung injury.

The neutrophil is the archetypal cell of an acute inflammatory response. Drawn in from the pulmonary capillaries by specific attractants, neutrophils too are well equipped to deal with microbes. They can produce a range of toxic free radicals and proteins, including enzymes such as elastase. The eosinophil also is capable of releasing a limited range of toxic mediators. However, it is only occasionally the prominent cell in acute pulmonary inflammation, typically asthma.

SPECIFIC DEFENCE

Macrophages and other cells, including dendritic fibroblasts, can present foreign material to lymphocytes triggering a more specific defensive response. Certain lymphocyte T-subsets are directly toxic to inhaled microbes. Others, the B-lymphocytes, create specific immunoglobulin (Ig) as antibody. Initially, IgM is secreted but later there is a switch to IgG and, in the lungs, IgA classes. The presence of one of these may be detected and used as a retrospective means of identifying the cause of an infective illness. Some vaccination techniques have been developed to elicit such a neutralising antibody response.

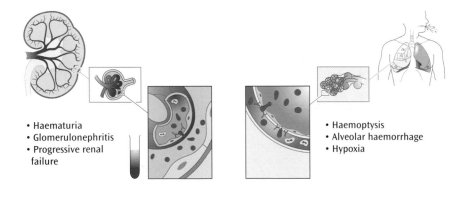

- Haematuria
- Glomerulonephritis
- Progressive renal failure

- Haemoptysis
- Alveolar haemorrhage
- Hypoxia

Fig. 2 **Goodpasture's syndrome – an example of a defence force (antibody) off target.** Antibodies are formed – for no clear reason – against a subunit of type IV collagen. This collagen is accessible to circulating antibody in both the glomerular and alveolar capillaries. Acute antibody driven inflammation occurs with damage and loss of membrane integrity.

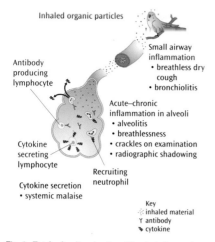

Fig. 3 **Extrinsic allergic alveolitis.** An inflammatory response – acute or chronic fibrosing – initiated by inhalation of organic material. Although predominantly pulmonary in pathology and symptoms, systemic effects may be masked.

cause inflammatory damage with loss of integrity and flooding of the alveoli with blood (alveolar haemorrhage). The deposits of antibody can be detected histologically.

Acute respiratory distress syndrome (ARDS)

ARDS describes the clinically severe end of a spectrum of lung injury that follows an often-recognised trigger to inflammation. The result is almost exclusively bystander damage that threatens the life of the host. Even with modern intensive care facilities, mortality of such acute lung injury is of the order of 50–70%. The trigger may be sepsis, trauma, massive blood transfusion or occasionally a combined or rare insult. Inflammation is triggered at capillary beds throughout the body including the pulmonary bed, which are often away from the site of the triggering stimulus. This inflammation involves many cell types but principally the neutrophil and macrophage/monocyte cells. As a result, the capillary endothelium becomes leaky with protein-rich fluid passing out into the

alveoli. This filling up of airspaces with non cardiogenic oedema results in hypoxaemia and bilateral infiltrates are seen on chest radiographs. Mechanical ventilatory support is often required, yet the stiff and poorly compliant lungs are not easy to ventilate and are susceptible to further damage by many ventilation strategies.

If the patient survives the initiating insult, hypoxia and the mechanical ventilation, then capillary integrity returns. The alveolar oedema becomes cellular early on and often undergoes a degree of fibrosis. Resolution takes many days. If there is a significant fibrotic component, clinical and radiological resolution may not be complete.

Current pulmonary therapy is entirely supportive and includes taking appropriate action against the trigger condition such as sepsis. Inhaled nitric oxide, acting as a local pulmonary vasodilator thereby increasing blood flow through parts of the lung that are ventilated, has been variously successful in ameliorating hypoxaemia. There is much current activity at identifying appropriate targets in the injurious inflammatory cascades and tissue recovery

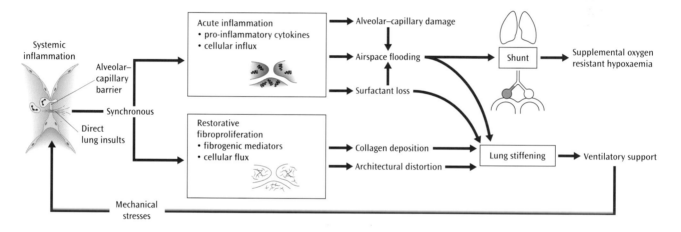

Fig. 4 **Acute lung injury: mechanisms and clinical consequences.**

DEFECTS OF HOST DEFENCE

Any element of the complex defence against inhaled foreign and potentially injurious materials may fail. An individual born with a defect of a major component is often severely compromised and it is often fatal. In contrast, a more minor disorder may lead only to repeated infections. Clinical awareness is required to identify individuals at most risk.

DISORDERED HOST DEFENCE

Goodpasture's syndrome

The formation of a circulating antibody is triggered by contact with an infection, possibly a chemical (Fig. 2). This antibody also identifies a component upon the glomerular capillary within the kidney. Interaction with it causes an inflammatory glomerulonephritis and risks impairing renal function. It also 'cross-reacts' with a component of the pulmonary capillary to

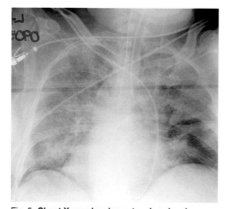

Fig. 5 **Chest X-ray showing extensive alveolar oedema of ARDS.**

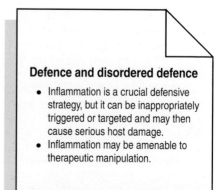

Defence and disordered defence

- Inflammation is a crucial defensive strategy, but it can be inappropriately triggered or targeted and may then cause serious host damage.
- Inflammation may be amenable to therapeutic manipulation.

THE CLINICAL HISTORY

Within most clinical medicine encounters, the history is the single most important aspect of the diagnostic process. Physical examination and subsequent investigations contribute proportionately less to the diagnostic process, but are clearly important in terms of confirmation, prognosis and therapy. Here follows a brief resume of the salient points that, without exception, should be explored in a respiratory history. It should be considered as complementary to, rather than substituting for, one of the many textbooks devoted to clinical history taking and examination.

MAJOR RESPIRATORY SYMPTOMS

The following are frequently the patient's main problem and should be gently explored. Allow them to tell you in their own manner, using a minimum of interruption and questioning to clarify important points.

Breathlessness

Difficulty with breathing or a sensation of inadequate breaths is probably the commonest and yet the most challenging of symptoms. It is termed dyspnoea. The perception results from a complex interplay between neuromuscular and cardiopulmonary sensations and the psyche. The causes may be respiratory but also cardiac, even metabolic, neuromuscular or psychological. Onset and duration must be fully characterised and the presence of other symptoms fully explored. Make an attempt at quantification by assessing either exercise capacity or tolerance and any disability. For example:

- Variable breathlessness over months or years may reflect airways obstruction or a recurrent cardiac tachy-dysrhythmia. The presence of subjective palpitations occurring before the breathlessness develops is the key to the latter which contrasts with associated cough, chest tightness and temporal association with temperature changes, dusty environments or other precipitants in asthma.
- Rapid onset of breathlessness over seconds to minutes is due to pneumothorax, pulmonary embolus, cardiac disease (usually a cardiac dysrhythmia) or in the context of 'shock'. Rarely can pneumococcal pneumonia present rapidly.
- Paroxysmal disturbance of sleep with breathlessness, cough and chest tightness should not be immediately equated with 'paroxysmal nocturnal dyspnoea' and hence left heart failure: it is often due to nocturnal exacerbations of asthma!
- Relentlessly progressive breathlessness without other respiratory symptoms is unusual but think of anaemia (source of blood loss?) and early interstitial lung disease with impaired lung compliance.
- Postural breathlessness is a feature of asthma and of left heart failure when breathlessness and distress is worse lying flat (orthopnoea). It is also a feature of diaphragmatic weakness with loss of gravitational assistance, especially noted when swimming.

Cough

Irritation of the nociceptive, usually non-myelinated fibres of the non-adrenergic non-cholinergic (NANC) pulmonary nervous system causes cough, which can be considered the central airways' sensory equivalent of pain. It arises as a symptom of mucosal inflammation or irritation. Features of the cough itself, the nature of any expectorated sputum and evidence of other cardiopulmonary symptoms should be sought. A change in the nature of a chronic cough should be considered as if it were new: patients with tobacco-induced chronic bronchitis may later develop a bronchial tumour.

A cough of infection may produce purulent sputum that is discoloured yellow-green. In the early stages of lobar pneumonia it may even be rust-coloured. Many viral infections are associated with a non-productive cough, and following pertussis infection in adults a protracted cough is sometimes a residua. Infected material dripping at night from chronically inflamed nasal sinuses into the oropharynx and larynx may be aspirated and expectorated the following day.

Non-infective causes of coughing include asthma. The eosinophil-rich airway inflammation may produce purulent-looking sputum as a result of eosinophil enzymes but without bacterial infection. The cough of asthma has a diurnal variability and other precipitants that are recognised exacerbating factors for asthma.

Irritation of central airways by tumour infiltration or the presence of an inhaled foreign body produces a new and often non-productive cough. These possibilities mandate bronchoscopic examination in patients with an otherwise unexplained cough, even if a chest radiograph is normal.

Haemoptysis

A cough productive of blood is an important and worrying symptom. The degree of blood produced may vary from streaking of sputum to clots. There are benign causes of haemoptysis, such as bronchiectasis where blood usually streaks purulent sputum or pulmonary infarction where clots can be expectorated. However, a bronchial malignancy must be the major clinical concern until proven otherwise, especially in a current or past cigarette smoker.

Chest pain

Chest wall muscular or skeletal (rib) pain is typically lateralised, sharp and made worse by coughing, deep breaths or on movement. It is worsened by direct pressure or by springing the thorax from a distance. The nature of the pain's onset is important, for example:

- a bout of vigorous coughing in an elderly person may be sufficient to cause a rib fracture
- the importance of eliciting a history of trauma is self-evident
- if gradual in onset may signify a viral myalgia (Bornholm disease).

Pleural pain is similar in so far as it is lateral and worsened by breathing and coughing. Such pleurisy is not typically worsened by twisting the trunk though there may be chest wall tenderness. The nature of its onset is very important. If sudden in onset, this raises the concerns of pulmonary embolism or a pneumothorax: a more gradual onset may be associated with other pleural pathologies and pleural fluid.

A deep-seated poorly localised hemi-thoracic ache is often associated with an ipsilateral malignancy or a large pleural effusion.

Nerve-root or intercostal nerve pain is knife-like in character as it radiates around the chest wall in a dermatomal distribution.

If recent onset it raises the possibility of herpes zoster infection (shingles) (Fig. 1), when the pain may appear a day or two before the diagnostic vesicular rash. Shingles pain is notoriously confusing and may initially be diagnosed as cardiac or pleuritic. Long-standing radicular pain may follow thoracotomy or be due to an intercostal neuroma.

Pain due to diaphragmatic irritation from lower thoracic or upper abdominal pathology is referred over the shoulder tip.

ADDITIONAL RESPIRATORY SYMPTOMS

These are often present and should be specifically sought in respiratory disease. They may be the presenting problem.

Hoarseness

Increased huskiness in a patient's voice may be due either to pathology local to the vocal cords (Fig. 2), such as tumour or benign thickening, or to disordered innervation. In the context of respiratory diseases, hoarseness is usually due to a malignant left recurrent laryngeal nerve palsy or a more generalised neuropathy such as motor neurone disease. A paralysed cord is unable to contain the intrathoracic pressure build-up of a normal cough response. The result is a weakened 'bovine' expectoration. Inhaled steroid use can cause huskiness as a result of local deposition.

Bone pain

Bone pain may reflect metastatic spread from a bronchial tumour. It must be confirmed and treated appropriately. Wrist pain and tenderness may represent the tender periosteal new bone formation of hypertrophic pulmonary osteo-arthropathy (HPOA) associated with rapidly progressive finger clubbing. Upper abdominal pain may represent liver capsule stretching either due to tricuspid valve incompetence in cor pulmonale or from metastatic tumour deposits. Hemi-facial pain is a rare feature of an ipsilateral pulmonary tumour and reflects vagal nerve involvement.

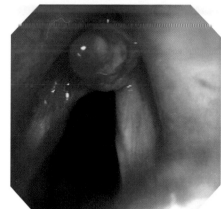

Fig. 2 **Vocal chord polyp is a cause of hoarseness.**

Weight loss

Weight loss is often a feature of malignancy. If not directly due to difficulty in swallowing, it is due to a combination of anorexia and tissue breakdown as part of a tumour-driven acute phase response. In severe chronic obstructive pulmonary disease, weight loss can be severe and impair both limb and respiratory muscle strength. In both disease processes there is usually a poor response to mere dietary manipulation. Weight gain may worsen both the upper airways obstruction and symptoms in obstructive sleep apnoea, and so precipitate medical attention.

IMPORTANT SOCIAL ELEMENTS

These are key features of any respiratory history.

- **Detailed smoking history.** Full details of age when started and quit, usual number smoked and maximum number smoked should be sought. Many 'non-smokers' are truly ex-smokers on further exploration.
- **Occupations.** A detailed chronological log from leaving school is required with an understanding of the job and likely exposures. The current job may be important to the patient's recent development of breathlessness. There may be exposure to some materials that are recognised to cause asthma or allergic alveolitis. Current respiratory disease may also be a legacy of exposure decades earlier (e.g. to asbestos).
- **Hobbies.** This may be as important as the workplace for inhaled material causing respiratory disease. Remember to enquire specifically about birds, including those of the neighbours!
- **Drugs.** Drugs such as β-blockers or non-steroidal anti-inflammatory agents (prescribed or purchased over a pharmacy counter) can worsen asthma. Rarely but devastatingly, some drugs induce lung disease. Treatment with prednisolone can reactivate, and newer antibiotics partially suppress, tuberculosis.

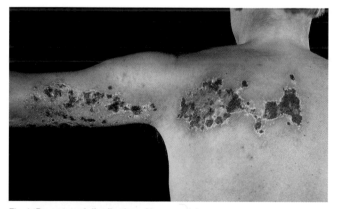

Fig. 1 **Dermatomal distribution of herpes zoster.**

Case history 4

An elderly lady with a recent diagnosis of late-onset asthma is referred up because she fails to respond to conventional inhaled therapy. Over 12 months she has noticed increasing breathlessness with an audible wheeze. This noise is worse at night, but seems to be eased when she leans forward. Weather, household fumes and smoky places do not appear to affect her symptoms in any way. Is this just asthma?

The clinical history

- Take time to explore fully the patient's presenting problems.
- Breathlessness can be a challenging symptom to determine the cause which may be far from cardiopulmonary in origin.
- Obtain a full and detailed occupational and cigarette smoking history.

PHYSICAL EXAMINATION I

The physical examination complements the history in the diagnostic process. It starts as soon as you first meet the patient: gait, degree of breathlessness and respiratory distress are noted. Similarly, exploring the history continues during the examination. This section offers a template and suggestions for performing a directed respiratory examination. However, it cannot replace learning and practising with an experienced clinician-educator.

It is usual to commence any physical examination with the patient's hands, moving in an orderly manner up to the head and neck then onto the trunk before finishing with the legs. Other systems of examination are equally valid. An introduction to the patient explaining what is about to happen is a minimal courtesy.

EXTRATHORACIC RESPIRATORY EXAMINATION

Hands
Examine both hands and all the fingers. Look for finger clubbing that ranges from loss of the nailfold angle to bulbous expansion of the fingertip (Fig. 1). There are many causes. Intrathoracic causes include:

- primary bronchial malignancy, usually non-small cell
- pulmonary fibrosis
- chronic sepsis as:
  – bronchiectasis: pus in the bronchi
  – empyema: pus in the pleural space
  – pulmonary abscess: pus in the lungs.

Pale warm hands may be a clue that the patient's breathlessness is due to anaemia. Blue discoloration, termed 'cyanosis', is usually due to increased

circulating desaturated haemoglobin. Rarely, it is due to an abnormal blood pigment such as methaemoglobin or a dye. Cold blue fingers are due to an inadequate peripheral circulation with increased oxygen extraction from the blood increasing desaturated haemoglobin: 'peripheral cyanosis'. Warm yet blue extremities are a feature of 'central cyanosis'. In this case good peripheral perfusion maintains warm fingers but the blood is inadequately oxygenated as a result of either severe respiratory disease or central mixing of oxygenated with deoxygenated mixed venous blood in a right-to-left shunt.

Examining the radial pulse may demonstrate the irregular rate and volume of atrial fibrillation. Supraventricular dysrhythmias are common in acute pulmonary conditions including infection, thromboembolism and acute or chronic respiratory failure, especially in the elderly. By causing a degree of cardiac decompensation, atrial fibrillation may contribute to or be the cause of breathlessness.

Wasting of muscle on the backs of the hand and thumb base may provide evidence of a generalised neuromuscular disorder or, if unilateral, a local nerve palsy.

Evidence of a vasculitis with nailfold infarcts and nail 'splinter haemorrhages' or an arthritis provide clues to the possible aetiology of a respiratory problem.

Arms
Scars and dust tattoos may reflect previous employment. Look for a BCG scar over the insertion site of the left deltoid muscle. Measure the systemic arterial blood pressure.

Head and neck
Warn patients before examining their face and neck. Is there conjunctival pallor of anaemia? The mouth and tongue may demonstrate Candida infection if the patient is debilitated and especially if mouth breathing. Blue discoloration of the warm mucosa under the tongue defines central cyanosis.

The jugular venous pulse wave should be examined. Elevated but pulsatile is in keeping with cor pulmonale or other right heart syndromes. Elevated but fixed with distended veins and

swelling over the neck and arms and conjunctival congestion are features of superior mediastinal obstruction (Fig. 2).

Enlargement of the parotid gland may reflect debility. It may be a feature of sarcoidosis if associated with a fever or, rarely, a unilateral facial nerve palsy.

Examine the neck for the position of the trachea which reflects the position of the upper mediastinum. Also assess the sternal angle-to-thyroid cartilage distance which is reduced to one or two finger breadths when the thorax is hyper-expanded.

The neck must be carefully examined from behind for lymph node enlargement. A flowing sequence of examination should include all node sites, the cervical chains, clavicular fossae and the scalenes.

Abdomen
There may be free abdominal fluid in cor pulmonale. A flattened diaphragm accompanying emphysema will allow a normal liver to be palpable in the abdomen. The clue that the liver is not enlarged is the displacement downwards of the upper border of liver dullness on percussion. Hepatic tenderness and enlargement with expansile pulsation are key features of tricuspid valve regurgitation that may reflect pulmonary hypertension. Hepatic pain, tenderness and craggy enlargement are all features of hepatic tumour deposits with liver capsule stretching.

Legs
Peripheral oedema accompanies cor

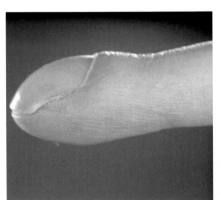
Fig. 1 **Finger clubbing and cyanosis.**

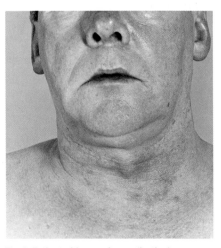
Fig. 2 **Patient with superior mediastinal obstruction.**

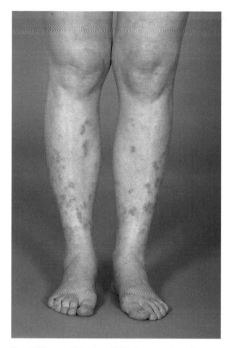

Fig. 3 **The pretibial purplish plaques of erythema nodosum.** This lady presented with the rash, painful ankles, a dry cough and hilar adenopathy on a chest radiograph.

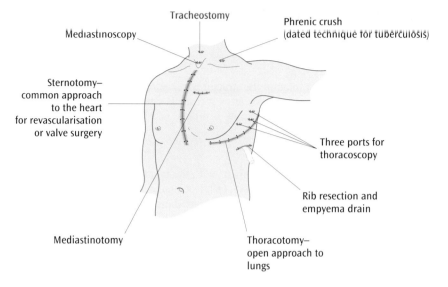

Fig. 4 **Scars commonly found on the thorax and their surgical implications.**

pulmonale. Unilateral or asymmetrical swelling should prompt serious consideration to the presence of deep venous thrombosis and hence of pulmonary thromboembolism.

Erythema nodosum is characterised by purplish painful plaques that develop over the legs, especially the shins, only to spontaneously subside over weeks (Fig. 3). This can be associated with streptococcal infections or be an acute presentation of sarcoidosis, especially in young women with bilateral hilar lymphadenopathy.

Toes as well as fingers may become clubbed.

THORACIC RESPIRATORY EXAMINATION

This should follow the traditional sequence of:

• inspection
• palpation
• percussion
• auscultation.

Inspection

Watch the patient from the end of the bed or the examination couch. What is the patient's respiratory rate and breathing pattern? Are they distressed resting or on the trivial exertion of undressing, or conversely can they complete a long-winded sentence with ease? Are they using their neck muscles as accessory muscles of inspiration? Is their breathing audible? Expiratory wheezes may be heard in severe airflow limitation: the harsh inspiratory noise of stridor indicates extrathoracic airway narrowing.

Are any scars present (Fig. 4)? Is the chest symmetrical? Regions of flattening particularly at the apex favours underlying pulmonary fibrosis.

Is chest expansion on both quiet and deep respiration equal and full? Any asymmetry of chest expansion immediately identifies the abnormal side in unilateral pathologies.

Indrawing or recession of the lower intercostal spaces in particular on inspiration is a feature of airflow limitation (Fig. 5). When severe, suprasternal sucking can be seen.

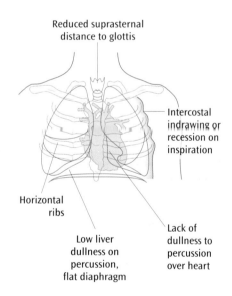

Fig. 5 **Hyper-expanded chest with intercostal recession of COPD.**

Case history 5

A 58-year-old gentleman presents with a 6-month history of exertion breathlessness without pains but with a nocturnal cough disturbing sleep. You wonder about asthma, but on examination the salient findings are a blood pressure of 165/60 with both ejection systolic and immediate diastolic cardiac murmurs audible. How is this relevant?

Physical examination 1

• Practice does improve skills!
• An orderly and thorough sequence of examination should be developed to become second nature.

PHYSICAL EXAMINATION II

SURFACE ANATOMY

When examining the chest, picture the structures beneath your fingers or stethoscope. Such knowledge of surface landmarks allows you to determine if the abnormality is limited to a lobe, for example (Fig. 1).

Palpation

The cardiac apex beat should be identified. With the trachea it identifies the position of the mediastinum. Displacement occurs in lobar or lung collapse, or in a tensioning pneumothorax.

The precordium should also be palpated for both the parasternal lift of right ventricle dilatation or hypertrophy and the thrill (palpable murmur) of pulmonary stenosis.

Chest expansion is best assessed by placing the fingertips on the skin, splayed symmetrically about the midline. The thumbs then act as calipers and their movement should be related to the midline (Fig. 2).

Percussion

The chest should be percussed moving symmetrically from the supraclavicular regions over the clavicle and down towards the abdomen, comparing left with right (Fig. 3). The lateral aspect of the thorax into the axillae should not be forgotten. The upper border of liver dullness on the right and the presence of cardiac dullness close to the lower left sternal edge should be specifically sought.

Pulmonary consolidation or collapse and pleural fluid will reduce the resonance of the percussion note. The stony dullness of pleural fluid, a complete lack of resonance upon percussion, can be imitated by percussing a solid wall.

The unilateral increased resonance of a pneumothorax may not be easily identified. Chest hyper-expansion is identified by signs other than bilaterally increased resonance.

Auscultation

Use the bell of the stethoscope to listen symmetrically over the chest, comparing left with right during quiet and then exaggerated respiration. Listen for the quality of the breath sounds and the presence of additional, abnormal sounds.

Normal breath sounds are quiet, predominantly inspiratory, with a noticeable pause before the quieter expiratory component. Assessment of the transmissibility of the thorax can be made by asking the patient to speak in a deep voice while auscultating over the lungs (vocal resonance). The word 'ninety-nine' is traditionally used as it encourages the lower frequencies. Consolidated lung will improve the audibility of the spoken word, whereas pleural fluid or thickening will diminish it. Attempt to assess the same qualities by palpation; 'tactile vocal fremitus' is less sensitive.

Bronchial breathing describes abnormally harsh breath sounds with equal inspiratory and expiratory noise: the cardinal physical sign of underlying pulmonary consolidation. It can be imitated by listening over the trachea. Indeed, transmission of tracheal noise can falsely suggest upper lobe consolidation when the trachea is deviated.

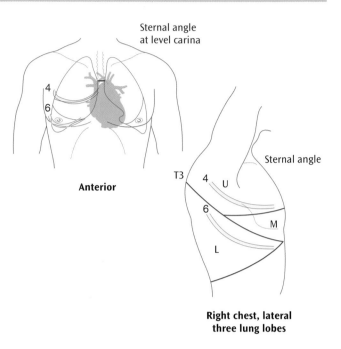

Fig. 1 **Surface positions of important thoracic levels and structures, in relation to fourth and sixth ribs.**

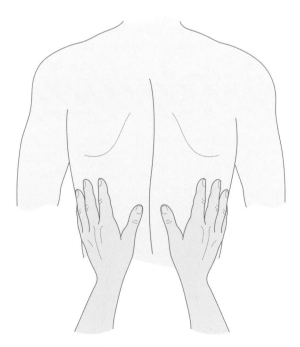

Fig. 2 **Examining for chest expansion.** The patient is making full respiratory excursions (vital capacity); the examiner's thumbs in the air act as calipers with respect to the spinous processes.

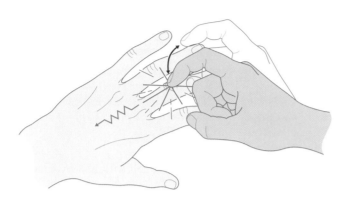

Fig. 3 **Technique of percussion:** percussing finger (wrist action) strikes finger or chest directly. Both sound and feeling generated are important.

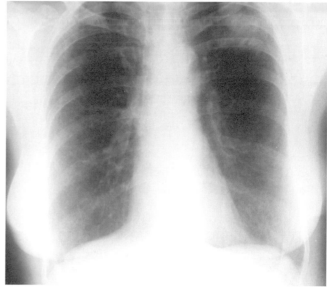

Fig. 4 **Chest radiograph as an extension of the physical examination.** The cause of this woman's malaise and weight loss was demonstrated by a radiograph, despite a normal chest examination.

	Consolidation	**Pneumothorax**	**Pleural fluid**	**Lobar collapse**	**Airways obstruction**
Thoracic signs					
Expansion	Reduced on right	Reduced on right	Reduced on left	Reduced on left	Symmetrical reduction
Percussion	Dull	Increased	Stone-like dullness	Dull but not stony	Resonant
Vocal fremitus	Increased	Absent	Absent	Reduced to absent with bronchial obstruction	Normal
Breath sounds	Harsh, bronchial breathing	Absent or reduced	Absent	Harsh if upper lobe as tracheal transmission	Vesicular
Added ?	Inspiratory crackles, possible rub	If left side, systolic click possible		Crackles often	Polyphonic wheezes
Extrathoracic features	Pleural pain Fever, sweats	Pleural pain		Double or straight edge to heart border on chest radiograph if left lower	Prolonged expiration Intercostal recession

Fig. 5 **Expected features on examination in common respiratory conditions.**

Added sounds consist of wheezes, crackles and rubs:

- *Wheezes* are continuous musical notes that are due to vibrations within the walls of airways usually as a result of their narrowing. When composed of several notes the term 'polyphonic' is used. Due to the narrower airway calibre on expiration, wheezes are more audible during, or may only be audible in, expiration. A 'fixed' monophonic wheeze that is invariable even after coughing suggests fixed bronchial obstruction, usually malignant.
- *Crackles* are discontinuous noises that are inspiratory and due to airspaces 'popping' open on inspiration. Traditionally much attention has been spent relating the nature and timing of crackles within the respiratory cycle to the underlying pathology but there is no evidence that any of these qualities allows such determination. Indeed some crackles originate from the pleura.
- *Pleural rubs* are typically variable, sounding rather creaky and said to be reminiscent of old leather. They reflect pleural inflammation.

Miscellaneous

The bedside measurement of peak expiratory flow rate or spirometry and the response to an inhaled bronchodilator could be considered part of the physical examination. Use of a pulse oximeter to measure transcutaneous oxygen saturation of arterial blood, and exhaled carbon monoxide estimation are also easily performed at the bedside and equally revealing. A chest radiograph is an extension of the physical examination, providing diagnostic information over and above that which could be obtained by examination alone (Fig. 4).

Physical examination II
- Practice does improve skills!
- A chest radiograph and spirometry are almost routine extensions of the clinical respiratory examination.

CLINICAL PRESENTATIONS OF RESPIRATORY DISEASE I

THE CHRONICALLY BREATHLESS PATIENT

The importance of a careful exploration of breathlessness and associated symptoms cannot be overemphasised. A detailed cardiopulmonary, thoracic and neuromuscular examination is usually required. Table 1 suggests a cardiopulmonary assessment. Many patients will have either asthma, or a combination of cardiac (ischaemic heart disease) and pulmonary (airways obstruction) causes contributing to exercise limitation.

Compared to respiratory exercise physiology testing, pulmonary function testing at rest is relatively insensitive to abnormalities, but often is all that is required. Patients with minimal symptoms, but nevertheless early respiratory disease, may have carbon monoxide gas transfer test results within the reference range, yet desaturated on exercise. By contrast, a patient who is unable to walk up stairs yet has a normal cardiopulmonary assessment will not have a respiratory or cardiac pathology as the sole cause for their exercise limitation. In the absence of cardiac murmurs, a normal resting 12-lead electrocardiogram (ECG) predicts good left ventricular performance and effectively excludes a dominant cardiac cause of limiting breathlessness.

Table 1 **Cardiopulmonary assessment**

Basic
Full clinical examination
Pulse oximetry or arterial blood gases (breathing air at rest)
Ventilatory capacity standing and lying
Resting 12-lead ECG
Chest radiograph
Full blood count
More detailed
Static lung volumes and gas transfer testing
Echocardiography
Respiratory exercise testing

Table 2 **The acutely breathless patient**

Initial resuscitation priorities
Are you and the patient safe?
Is the patient responsive? Gently shake and shout at the patient
Open and maintain an airway
Is the patient breathing? Look, listen and feel for chest movement and airflow at the mouth for no more than 10 seconds
Does the patient have a heart beat? Feel a neck pulse for no more than 10 seconds
Initial clinical assessment
Respiratory and heart rate
Ability to converse? Confused?
Tracheal position
Chest expansion symmetrical
Pulse oximetry, peak flow, cardiac rhythm monitor
Effectiveness of peripheral circulation
Concomitant initial therapeutic manoeuvres
Deliver high flow oxygen
Place a large bore intravenous cannula

Beware of pericardial fluid, however.

Neuromuscular causes of breathlessness are unusual and often overlooked. Exercise limitation and subjective breathlessness due to motor neurone disease is often associated with voice or swallowing difficulties and muscle wasting with fasciculation on examination. Seemingly unrelated past events, such as a whiplash neck injury in a road traffic accident or the earache of herpes zoster, may provide the clue to phrenic nerve injury, diaphragmatic palsy and undue breathlessness. Imaging the diaphragms by radiography or ultrasound while the patient is sniffing should confirm paralysis. A more general test of respiratory neuromuscular integrity is postural spirometry (Fig. 1).

Breathlessness unrelated to the degree of activity performed is a clue to the hyperventilation syndrome. Patients may admit to being unable to take a 'big enough breath in'. This breathlessness is often associated with chest pains and with dysaesthesia of the extremities as neuromuscular function is disturbed by the respiratory alkalosis. Cardiopulmonary disease may be present, but the breathlessness is out of proportion to the dysfunction. A provocation test of 20 hyperventilation breaths may reproduce the symptoms, though a formal exercise test is sometimes required to demonstrate ventilation out of proportion to the workload (Fig. 2). An empathic explanation to the patient is required so the diagnosis is accepted before breathing retraining can commence.

Being substantially overweight can of itself be a cause of chronic breathlessness, often with an associated lack of cardiopulmonary fitness. Increasing weight can cause increasing breathlessness; other features such as cough are not to be expected. Typically, there is the apparent paradox of breathlessness and limitation performing weight-bearing exercise, but with a better performance when not weight bearing. Significant breathlessness is not to be expected unless the individual's body mass index (weight/(height)^2) is substantially over 30.

THE ACUTELY BREATHLESS PATIENT

Rapid assessment of the patient using the basic principles of resuscitation is the first priority (Table 2). The ABC of airway, breathing and circulation should be supplemented with a rapid clinical assessment (Table 2). Assessment with therapy continues and close clinical review maintained as diagnostic possibilities are explored:

- **Respiratory** – pneumothorax, pulmonary emboli, acute asthma, anaphylaxis.
- **Cardiovascular** – pulmonary oedema, myocardial infarction , dysrhythmia.
- **Miscellaneous** – shock, hypovolaemic or anaphylactic, occasionally septic.

CHEST PAIN

Chest pain is a common problem and not always respiratory in origin; cardiac and oesophageal conditions are common. Sometimes and despite much searching, the cause of the pain may not be evident. In this case, effective analgesia and continued observation is prudent.

PLEURISY

Lateralised chest wall pain that is worsened by coughing or breathing is a common symptom. A directed history and

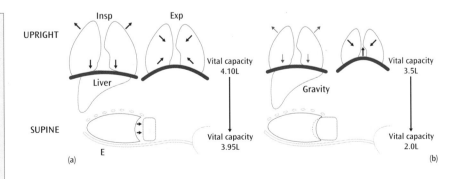

Fig. 1 **Neuromuscular weakness and postural decrement vital capacity. (a)** Normal respiratory muscle strength. **(b)** Clinically significant respiratory muscle weakness results in a small vital capacity and total lung capacity measured upright. When supine the now added load of the abdominal content is not overcome and lung volumes are even smaller. When in water this loading is even greater.

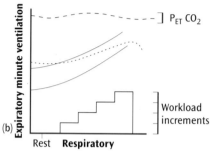

(a)

Note: Normal haemodymanic response to exercise

(b)

Minute ventilation at rest exceeds predicted, as exercise load increases becomes as predicted with expired CO_2 pattern similarly normalising during exercise. This is the pattern seen in hyperventilation syndrome

Fig. 2 **Results from cardiopulmonary exercise testing. (a)** Cardiovascular; **(b)** respiratory.

examination are essential. The nature of the onset of pain, and any associated respiratory symptoms and signs, is important. A chest radiograph is necessary. A pneumothorax should be carefully looked for, as well as features of pulmonary infarction or pleuropulmonary infection. Further investigation and additional imaging may be required.

MUSCULOSKELETAL CHEST WALL PAIN

Musculoskeletal pathology can cause pleural pain that is worse on movement. Rib fractures following coughing, trauma or a bone metastasis will present with localised and reproducible rib tenderness. Muscular causes may have similar exami-

nation findings. Pulmonary infarction, or infection, can also cause chest wall tenderness. Burning, uncomfortable, neuralgic pain that shoots around the trunk may precede the eruption of a blistering rash diagnostic of shingles!

Lateral chest wall pain

This is pain that is neither typically pleuritic nor musculoskeletal. Processes that need to be considered include tumour infiltration into the chest wall. This tends to cause a relentless pain, poorly relieved by modest analgesics. Lancinating pain that shoots around the chest may be referred from spinal pathology including vertebral fracture but it may also be the presentation of a rare neural tumour, an intercostal nerve neuroma.

Central chest pain

Pain that is ischaemic or cardiac in origin is the commonest concern. This is typically heavy or pressing, described with non-verbal indications of tightness or pressure. Features of autonomic system disturbance including sweating and nausea with undue breathlessness are common associations. Electrocardiograph changes may be absent.

Similarly severe and unpleasant pains can occur in a number of other conditions, often with subtle features that provide the clue to diagnosis. In massive pulmonary emboli a feeling of faintness or collapse is likely. An aortic tear is often associated with midback pain. The pain of spontaneous oesophageal rupture is often just preceded by the patient retching or trying not to vomit. A strangulating hiatus hernia is rare but a chest radiograph is of great assistance (Fig. 3).

COUGH AND SPUTUM PRODUCTION

Many patients are troubled by and present to medical care with a productive cough (Fig. 4). The length of time the cough has been present, the appearance of sputum

expectorated and the presence of any associated cardiorespiratory or systemic features need to be established.

Recent onset of cough with breathlessness or fevers and malaise would suggest a lower respiratory tract infection. The sputum may be discoloured or even rust-brown in appearance. Associated symptoms may include pleurisy, rigors, confusion or gastrointestinal upset.

Recurrent or repeated episodes of cough and discoloured sputum suggest bronchiectasis or asthma. The presence of pleurisy or haemoptysis may occur in the former and wheezy chest tightness with the latter. However, neither may be prominent or present. Some patients with asthma receive a number of courses of antibiotics until the diagnosis is reached and airway inflammation causing sputum production is suppressed.

A daily cough productive of clear sputum, perhaps with periods of discoloration, would suggest chronic irritation from inhaled irritants as in chronic bronchitis due to tobacco smoke exposure.

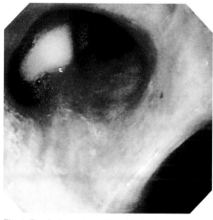

Fig. 4 **Pus in bronchus.** Bronchiectasis was confirmed radiologically.

Case history 6

A middle-aged smoker describes severely limiting breathlessness due to asbestosis-induced lung disease and is pursuing a legal action. Examination of his heart and lungs is normal. His resting lung function is measured and is normal. He struggles to complete a treadmill exercise test, stopping at half target workload due to breathlessness. However, on a separate occasion he completes satisfactorily another bicycle exercise test.

Comment?

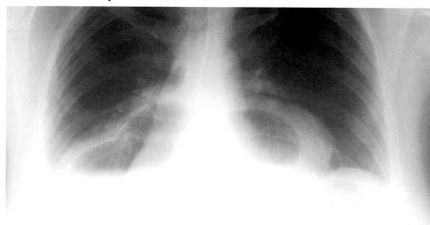

Fig. 3 **Hiatus hernia seen on chest radiograph.** Her pain was due to strangulation and subsequent gangrene.

CLINICAL PRESENTATIONS OF RESPIRATORY DISEASE II

CHRONIC COUGH

The most important features to explore are the nature of the onset and whether the cough has persisted relentlessly since onset or if there is any variability, with precipitants or associated symptoms.

Post-viral bronchial hyper-reactivity

A cough that has persisted following an upper respiratory tract viral infection may well represent post-viral bronchial hyper-reactivity. Look for variability, both diurnal and following exposures that typically worsen asthma. There may be associated wheeze, or a past or family history of atopy. Physical examination may be normal without evidence of air-

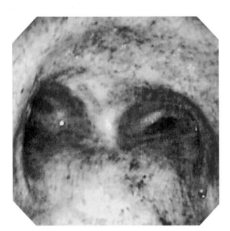

Fig. 1 **Diffusely inflamed bronchial mucosa in a patient with a persistent cough and chest tightness due to (at time of bronchoscopy) untreated asthma.**

ways obstruction, though measuring a peak flow rate often brings on a bout of coughing. A course of oral prednisolone should produce an impressive improvement and the benefit is maintained by inhaled steroids (Fig. 1). So important is this diagnosis, and so gratifying to treat effectively, that I have a low threshold for such a steroid trial.

Chronic rhino-sinusitis

Similar patients may also have chronic sinus inflammation with nasal stuffiness, blockage and catarrh. Mucus dripping posteriorly into the nasopharynx may be aspirated at night and may cause a nocturnal or early morning cough that must be differentiated from bronchial hyper-reactivity.

Cardiac failure

Cardiac failure also causes a predominantly nocturnal cough, though usually with exertional breathlessness. Examination will demonstrate inspiratory crackles at both lung bases, a triple heart rhythm and, possibly, a cardiac murmur. A common clinical problem is the patient with known cardiac disease and a persistent irritating cough. This may represent pulmonary venous engorgement when venodilators, such as nitrates, are particularly helpful. More likely the patient is taking an angiotensin converting enzyme inhibitor (ACEI); cough is a recognised side-effect. I find the frequency of ACEI-induced cough overestimated. The majority of patients will tolerate their cough once they have been reminded of the undoubted survival benefits of such therapy.

Reflux

Though gastro-oesophageal reflux and micro-aspiration of gastric acid into the lungs can cause coughing, confirmation is difficult. Upper gastrointestinal endoscopy is unhelpful and facilities for ambulatory oesophageal pH monitoring are not widely available. Though many patients have reflux symptoms that may be coincidental, a therapeutic trial of effective acid suppression is often undertaken.

Infections

Bordetella pertussis infection in non-immune adults is on the increase, not just in the cohort of 1970s children who missed vaccination because of an encephalopathy scare. Whooping cough in adults can be chronic and the diagnosis needs serological confirmation. Tuberculosis rarely presents as an isolated cough without other clinical or radiological signs.

Tumours

Though a chest radiograph may demonstrate a proximal tumour, an undiagnosed cough requires bronchoscopic examination of the central airways for tumour (Fig. 2), inhaled foreign body (Fig. 3) or other bronchial abnormality. Bronchial washings can also be taken for culture and examined for eosinophils.

Idiopathic

Once these investigations and diagnoses have been considered, to no avail, one is often left with a patient with a chronic cough that is worsened in public places or with anxiety. There is increasing experience and success with regular oral cap-

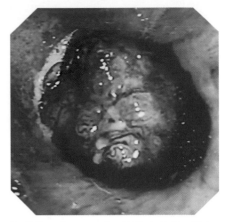

Fig. 2 **Bronchoscopy view of airway tumour in a patient who presented with a 9-week history of intractable cough.** He was a smoker, yet chest radiograph was normal.

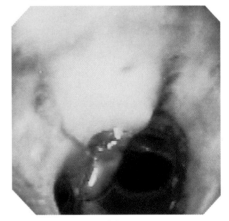

Fig. 3 **Inhaled coal particle.**

saicin present in a confectionery lozenge. This is said to have the effect of chronically stimulating, and thereby depleting, neurotransmitter substance P stores within NANC nerve fibres to interrupt the neural pathway of the cough reflex.

HAEMOPTYSIS

The most important diagnostic elements are:

- Is blood truly coughed up? The volume of blood does not discriminate between a respiratory or gastrointestinal origin. Life-threatening haemoptyses are often initially considered a haematemesis. Nosebleeds rarely bleed solely posteriorly, so associated epistaxis makes a nasal source very likely. The appearances of any sputa associated with the blood can help. Purulent sputum suggests a lower respiratory tract infection but haemoptysis should never be attributed solely to infection unless other causes have

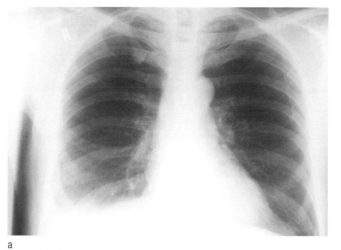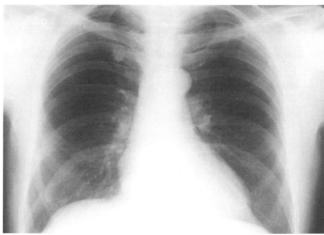

a   b

Fig. 4 **Coincidental finding. (a)** Unexpected radiograph finding of pleural fluid and a fractured rib. An appropriate history confirmed substantial thorax trauma 2 months previously. A follow-up film **(b)** shows spontaneous resolution of the pleural fluid has occurred.

been fully considered.

- Has the haemoptysis been occurring intermittently over years, perhaps with pleurisy and sputum purulence, suggesting bronchiectasis?
- Is there associated pleurisy or pain making pulmonary infarction a concern?
- Is there evidence of a bleeding diathesis or coagulopathy? Haemoptysis is an uncommon presentation but some coagulopathies, such as von Willebrand's disease, may present in adult life.

In the absence of an alternative diagnosis, a flexible bronchoscopy is indicated even if a chest radiograph is normal, whether or not the patient smokes. Being a current or ex-smoker makes an underlying tumour more likely, but it should not be a diagnosis excluded on the basis of 'never smoked'. Non-malignant possibilities include benign bronchial carcinoid, adenoma or inhaled foreign body (Fig. 3). CT lung scanning is also important in the investigation of a patient with otherwise unexplained haemoptysis. A high resolution scan is more sensitive than a plain chest radiograph in identifying bronchiectasis. If performed before bronchoscopy, and a localised abnormality is demonstrated, particular attention can then be paid to the area in question.

ABNORMAL CHEST RADIOGRAPH

A chest radiograph often performed with other reasons in mind may turn up an abnormality completely unrelated to the indication: a coincidental finding. The most rewarding way to proceed is to enquire about and retrieve previous such radiographs for comparison. Indeed,

obtaining previous chest films to compare with the current is a valuable 'investigation' in its own right. Previous films may be lodged elsewhere, performed for reasons that might include insurance medical examinations or pre-employment screening. Unfortunately, many old films are destroyed due to lack of storage space. The radiologist's report may be sufficiently helpful but often is never the same as inspecting the films for oneself. Such comparison can give an idea of rate of change, if any, in the abnormality.

A review of past events with the patient is also required. A fall, chest trauma or previous illness or employment may provide the required information (Fig. 4). Further evaluation is then required, depending on the abnormality and tailored to the individual.

LEG SWELLING

Unilateral leg swelling is significant for respiratory disease. It raises clinical concern of venous thrombosis and, hence, of pulmonary emboli. However, clinical suspicion is insufficient and should be confirmed by further investigation.

Bilateral and symmetrical leg swelling or oedema is a feature of cor pulmonale and hypoxaemic respiratory failure. It can be transiently present during an exacerbation of COPD. However, such leg oedema can be similarly present in congestive cardiac failure and other states with salt and fluid retention, including chronic liver disease and nephrosis, or lymphoedema. One of the commonest causes is dependency due to poor mobility.

Case history 7

A 65-year-old smoker without current respiratory symptoms has a chest radiograph performed following a new diagnosis of hypertension. He is referred urgently for investigation of a pleural effusion with a concern of malignancy. Figure 4a reproduces that radiograph.

Comments?

Clinical presentations of respiratory disease II

- A normal resting 12-lead ECG in the absence of cardiac murmurs predicts preserved left ventricular function.
- Postural spirometry is a simple, but effective, way of assessing respiratory neuromuscular function.
- Breathlessness unrelated to the degree of effort? Think of the hyperventilation syndrome, diagnose positively and manage with empathy and support.
- Bronchoscopy is indicated whenever there is a new or changed cough, as well as following haemoptysis, even if a chest radiograph is normal.

UPPER AND LOWER RESPIRATORY TRACT INFECTIONS

UPPER RESPIRATORY TRACT INFECTIONS

These are a group of mainly viral infections.

COMMON COLD

The common cold refers to acute symptoms, including nasal stuffiness and runniness, sore throat, sneezing, blocked ears, runny eyes and fever, that last for 1–2 days. It can be caused by any one of a number of respiratory viruses including adenoviruses, entero- and rhino-viruses and the influenza and parainfluenza viruses. Secondary bacterial infection, especially in patients with underlying cardiorespiratory conditions, contributes to morbidity.

INFLUENZA

Influenza is a prostrating systemic viral infection with muscle aches, arthralgia and headache in association with fevers and nasal congestion, sore throat, ears or eyes which may last for many days. It is highly infectious, transmitted by nasal droplets and caused by influenza viruses that undergo frequent mutation. Most epidemics occur in winter with world-wide pandemics due to major surface antigen mutations occurring most decades. Morbidity and mortality are significant, especially at the extremes of age and in patients with underlying chronic disease. Secondary bacterial infection commonly adds to the mortality. Vaccination of people most at risk may reduce both mortality and the effect of epidemics (Fig. 1).

CROUP

Croup (laryngo-tracheo-bronchitis) may follow symptoms of a cold in young children with breathlessness and stridor that can last for several days. The respiratory distress is alarming but responds well to steam inhalations and nebulised or oral steroids. It may recur with subsequent infections.

ACUTE EPIGLOTTITIS

Acute epiglottitis is a potentially life-threatening infection of the epiglottis with resultant swelling and airway compromise caused by capsulated *Haemophilus influenzae* type b. It is now rare in young children in the UK due to an effective vaccination programme, but sporadic cases still occur in non-immune children and adults. The illness usually starts mildly, with fever and sore throat, but can progress rapidly with voice changes to respiratory distress and stridor. Prompt antibiotic therapy is necessary, but skilled invasive airway management with intubation or tracheostomy may be required (Fig. 2).

DIPHTHERIA

Diphtheria too is now uncommon in developed countries due to effective vaccination. It can cause stridor with an inflammatory membrane visible on the pharynx and a bloody nasal discharge. Systemic effects, including myocarditis, are due to a toxin. Penicillin and immune serum are effective.

LOWER RESPIRATORY TRACT INFECTIONS

TRACHEITIS AND TRACHEOBRONCHITIS

Infection causes retrosternal chest pain with rawness on breathing. There is often a dry cough or a cough productive of scant purulent secretions. Systemic upset is rare except at the extremes of age. Focal physical signs on chest examination are absent. Adenoviruses are the most common pathogens but others include the 'flu viruses, enteroviruses, even measles. Analgesia and an anti-tussive may be required.

Whooping cough is a specific form of bacterial tracheobronchitis with airway mucosal inflammation and necrosis caused by *Bordetella pertussis*. Patients present with a runny nose and dry cough that may lead to paroxysms of coughing followed by an inspiratory 'whoop'. Upper thoracic petechiae may occur, secondary bacterial infection is common and encephalitis is rare.

ACUTE PURULENT BRONCHITIS

Secondary bacterial infection may complicate viral infections. Pathogens include non-encapsulated *H. influenzae*, staphylococci and streptococci. Patients will have a cough productive of purulent secretions with a fever. Auscultation will reveal noises consequent on secretions moving in the large airways. Simple analgesia, adequate hydration and assistance with expectoration of viscid purulent secretions may be required. Antibiotics are traditionally prescribed. Recurrent bouts of bronchitis in children should prompt consideration of an immune deficiency or cystic fibrosis, in adults that of asthma.

BRONCHOPNEUMONIA

This is an infection that can range in clinical severity from a short-lived episode in an otherwise young, healthy person to a life-threatening, if not life-terminating, illness in elderly patients with other major diseases. Bacteria or viruses may be responsible. Patients are ill, febrile and breathless, with a cough usually productive of purulent secretions. Examination reveals focal crackles. There are clinical similarities with pneumonia but pleural pain and bronchial breath sounds are absent. Antibiotics, physiotherapy with humidification, oxygen and hydration may be required. Bronchopneumonia is often the cause of death of patients with other serious underlying diseases.

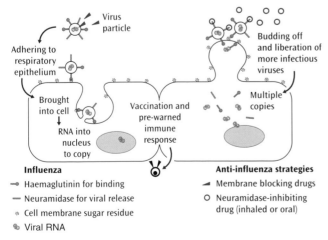

Fig. 1 **Influenza replication and antiviral strategies.**

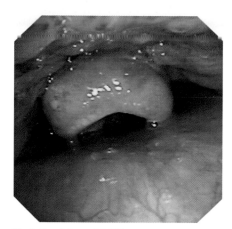

Fig. 2 **Resolving epiglottitis.**

PNEUMONIA

Pneumonia is still a major cause of death world-wide. In many developing countries it is the commonest cause of death from infectious disease. In the UK more patients die yearly from pneumonia than from asthma. Case fatality rates fell following the introduction of penicillin, but have failed to fall much further, currently around 10–25%. Many patients with pneumonia and lower respiratory tract infections are very appropriately managed in primary care, one of the commonest reasons for attending and for prescribing. About 1% are referred onward to hospital.

Classification

Pneumonia classifications have previously been based on microbiological causes or on the concept of clinically typical (pneumococcal) pneumonia and atypical pneumonia such as *Legionella* or mycoplasma. Since there are no clinico-radiological features unique for any particular microbiological cause, pneumonia should be classified clinically as:

- community-acquired pneumonia
- nosocomial or hospital-acquired pneumonia, clinically arising 48 hours or more after hospital admission
- aspiration pneumonia, with chemical and infectious lung injury
- pneumonia in an immuno-compromised host
- tuberculosis.

Pathology

Inhaled microbes are deposited on the respiratory epithelium and are met by the surface phagocytes. Host defence by local epithelial cells and phagocytes escalates to an archetypal acute inflammatory response. The balance between injury, host defence and infection determines the clinical picture and outcome.

Driven by inflammation-promoting chemicals (cytokines), the local vessels engorge, and a protein-rich plasma exudate seeps out to flood the alveoli. Circulating neutrophils adhere to, and migrate between, the endothelial cells into the interstitium and out into the alveoli to support resident macrophages in microbe killing and neutralisation. This inflammatory and cellular exudate fills the pulmonary segment, or lobe, and becomes organised into a firm solid material, termed hepatisation. The clinical and radiological equivalent is consolidation.

If this defence continues successfully, the pathogenic bacteria and toxic chemicals are neutralised. Resolution occurs with removal of debris. Streptococci typically elicit an inflammatory response that occurs without resulting lung damage. Other bacteria, staphylococci and Gram-negative bacteria cause substantial lung cell death with resolution to abnormal architecture.

Associated with this local inflammatory response, there is a systemic inflammatory reaction with changes in other vascular beds driven by circulating cytokines and cells. Many of these changes are clinically silent, but may become apparent as acute lung injury, abnormal liver or gastrointestinal function, as well as with vascular disturbances.

Clinical features

Symptoms usually include cough and undue breathlessness, fever and malaise. Any cough is initially non-productive as the inflammatory material is not freely mobile. Pleural pain may be prominent, especially in young people. Extrapulmonary manifestations, including diarrhoea and skin rash, may be the reason for presentation.

Examination may note an ill, feverish person, perhaps with a lip cold sore. Both heart and respiratory rate with a blood pressure should be noted. Atrial fibrillation commonly accompanies infection in elderly patients; an uncontrolled ventricular response may cause additional pulmonary oedema and cardiac ischaemia. Oxygenation should be measured by pulse oximetry.

Chest examination will usually demonstrate the signs of pulmonary consolidation. Sometimes the physical signs are relatively slight or conversely extensive and bilateral.

A chest radiograph will demonstrate opacification of the lung segments involved which may be lobar or more patchy. This lags behind the development of clinical symptoms and signs so a

very early radiograph may demonstrate minimal changes. A reverse contrast effect of air filling bronchi with surrounding airspace consolidation is termed an 'air bronchogram' (Fig. 3). This radiological sign of consolidation should be sought. A marked discrepancy between scant physical signs and extensive radiological abnormality is more likely to occur in tuberculosis or mycoplasma infections. Resolution of these radiological changes lags well behind clinical response to treatment and may take months to clear, especially in patients who are elderly or with pre-existing lung abnormalities, including proximal bronchial obstruction by tumour.

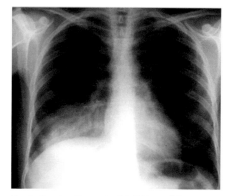

Fig. 3 **Chest radiograph of right lower lobe consolidation with an air bronchogram.**

Case study 8

A 35-year-old mother presents with a sore throat over several days but now with increasing hoarseness and noisy breathing. What is your concern?

Upper and lower respiratory tract infections

- There are a range of organisms that can cause upper respiratory infections. Many are trivial but may be devastating to patients at the extremes of age or with co-existing disease.
  A few may be prevented by effective vaccination.
- The most useful approach to pneumonia utilises a clinically based classification rather than contrasting perceived typical with non-typical infections.

PNEUMONIA

COMMUNITY-ACQUIRED PNEUMONIA (CAP)

Bacteriology

Streptococcus pneumoniae is the commonest pathogen. Studies that have specifically sought the microbiological cause of pneumonia, utilising antigen detection methods, suggest that it may cause up to 70% of cases. Although it typically causes a lobar pneumonia, patchy radiological infiltration may occur. In countries as diverse as Papua New Guinea and Spain, pneumococci are becoming resistant to penicillin.

Staphylococcus aureus is an unusual cause of pneumonia, but can be lethal when complicating influenza infection. Patients with a preceding 'flu-like illness' or who are admitted from residential care where such viral infections spread rapidly require antibiotics that will cover staphylococci. Methicillin-resistant strains may cause community-acquired pneumonia.

Legionella pneumophilia was identified as a new pulmonary pathogen after an outbreak of severe pneumonia at a convention of the American Legion in 1976. Since then there have been further outbreaks, some provoking media attention, and sporadic cases. Though it causes only 2–10% of hospitalised pneumonia cases, it is responsible for over 30% of those admitted to critical care areas. It is a pathogen that flourishes in environmental warm water and such sources of infection include showers, air-conditioning units and cooling towers. This organism is resistant to penicillins, but macrolides and rifampicin are effective. The presence of the organism can be sought directly on pulmonary specimens, or by antigen excretion in the urine. A rise in serum-specific antibody can take up to 6 weeks.

Other bacteria causing primary community-acquired pneumonia are rare, but include *Klebsiella* and other Gram-negative pathogens.

Mycoplasma pneumoniae is an unusual cause of hospitalisation. It occurs in 3-yearly autumnal epidemics and sporadic outbreaks. A persistent, dry cough, occasionally with rash and earache, occur. Clinical signs are often less than a radiograph would suggest. The production of cold agglutinins against an erythrocyte surface antigen (I antigen) may occur and cause haemolysis. Confirmation of the diagnosis is an early rise in serum IgM-specific antibody.

Macrolides or tetracycline are required for therapy.

Chlamydia psittaci may be caught from psittacine birds, such as parrots, to cause pneumonia, meningo-encephalitis or even hepatitis. Confirmation is serological and retrospective, yet effective treatment requires tetracycline or a macrolide. Cats, now the commonest pet in the UK, may be a reservoir for feline *Chlamydia psittaci*.

Chlamydia pneumoniae is a recently recognised pathogen. Epidemiological studies have demonstrated frequent subclinical infection before adulthood, in addition to clinical epidemics. There is increasing interest in a link with atherosclerosis.

Coxiella burnetti is an obligate intracellular microbe that was first recognised following an epidemic of pneumonia in Queensland, termed Q-fever. It is mainly an occupational infection of farming, veterinary and abattoir workers typically affecting workers in springtime. Treatment is with tetracyclines.

Viral infections are rarely associated with radiographic dense lobar consolidation, more usually patchy and often bilateral, a 'pneumonitis'. However, infections can be severe, superinfection with bacteria a cause of mortality and person-to-person spread a real risk. Primary measles pneumonitis with secondary bacterial infection is a common cause of childhood mortality and morbidity in the developing world. Respiratory syncitial (RSV) infection is common among children under 5 years during the winter months. Adults may occasionally suffer a severe illness. The bronchiolitis and pneumonitis is often associated with a wheeze that may persist. Bronchial secretions need to be specifically examined for viral antigen as serological studies are of necessity retrospective. Specific therapy is lacking for many, but antiviral agents for RSV and herpes simplex and varicella-zoster are available (Fig. 1).

Clinical management

Treatment and investigations begin as soon as a clinical and radiological diagnosis of community-acquired pneumonia has been made. A chest radiograph is essential as clinical judgement may be wrong. Specific antimicrobial therapy must commence as soon as the diagnosis is made, before admission to hospital and well before the results from initial investigations are available. The choice of

antibiotics is determined by severity of illness and local experience, but must include cover for *Strep. pneumoniae*. Additionally, cover for *Staphylococcus* must be included during 'flu epidemics, for mycoplasma in epidemic years and for *Legionella* if severe. There are many guidelines with appropriate antibiotics suggested. Thereafter, therapy is modified in the light of microbiological results. Non-specific aspects of therapy include pain-relief for pleurisy, oxygen and fluid balance.

In hospital practice initial useful investigations include blood and sputum samples for culture and pneumococcal antigen testing (Fig. 2). A serum sample should be obtained for mycoplasma IgM testing in an epidemic year and reserved for later testing against a convalescent sample for rising titres. In community medical practice it is often impractical to consider any initial routine microbiological sampling.

Severity, morbidity and mortality

Several basic clinical parameters have been validated in large scale studies as important markers of severity:

1. confusion, cyanosis and co-morbidities
2. respiratory rate >30 per minute
3. diastolic blood pressure <60 mmHg
4. blood urea >7.0 mM.

The presence of two or three of the above predicts a group of patients with a 21-fold risk of mortality and includes 95% of those who subsequently die from CAP. Such simple criteria should be used in policies for hospital admission, antibiotic therapy and even critical care support. Patients requiring critical care support tend to be younger and previously well, yet mortality rates are high, approaching 50%. The range of

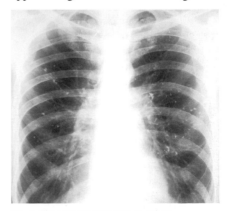

Fig. 1 **Chest radiograph with flecks of calcification in lungs of healed chickenpox pneumonitis.**

pathogens is similar, but *Legionella* is responsible for about 30%.

Morbidity is substantial, with a median 11 days in hospital. A quarter of patients will not have returned to normal activities by 6 weeks.

Mortality from CAP occurs either within a day or two from hypoxia, or later from multi-organ failure. The late administration of inappropriate antibiotics contributes.

Treatment failure

If a patient with pneumonia fails to respond to therapy then consider:

- **Is the diagnosis right?** Pulmonary emboli and pulmonary vasculitis can both cause pulmonary consolidation with systemic upset including fever. If the patient requires mechanical ventilation then there may be the opportunity to obtain invasive samples for microbiological and pathological investigation, by either bronchoscopy or lung biopsy.
- **Are the antibiotics appropriate?** Adding more antibiotics without thought is unhelpful, but is *Legionella* or another uncommon pathogen possible, and is it being adequately covered? Could aspiration be occurring with differing microbiology? Is it tuberculosis?
- **Is there a complication of the illness or therapy?** Penicillins can cause fever. An associated pleural empyema can develop with persistent fever requiring early recognition, vigorous drainage and possible surgical intervention. Is the pneumonia secondary to bronchial obstruction by tumour or inhaled foreign body, or is an abscess developing?

NOSOCOMIAL PNEUMONIA

Hospital-acquired pneumonia

Hospital-acquired pneumonia is caused by differing organisms from community infections, and antibiotics chosen must reflect this. Gram negative bacilli are more common, pneumococci are possible and *Legionella* is an important cause in terms of illness severity and socio-environmental implications.

Ventilator-associated pneumonia

Ventilator-associated pneumonia is a particular type of nosocomial infection occurring in critically ill patients, often with many other potential causes for fever, leucocytosis and radiological lung infiltrates. Direct sampling of the lower airway is often necessary since culture of tracheal secretions can be misleading. Infecting bacteria often originate from the gastrointestinal tract. Bacteria colonise the stomach and micro-aspiration occurs past the endotracheal tube cuff into the lungs. Achieving gastric acidity for a period in each 24 hours prevents gastric colonisation by bacteria and may reduce pulmonary infections.

ASPIRATION PNEUMONIA

A number of patients are at risk of aspiration pneumonia. This includes those who:

- are stuporosed or unconscious, rarely following anaesthesia
- have swallowing difficulties from any cause, may inhale while attempting to swallow. A local oesophageal abnormality, such as stricture or hiatus hernia, may allow material to collect only to be inhaled when asleep (Fig. 3).

All are at risk of inhaling either potentially infected vomitus or passively regurgitated material into their lungs. This can happen acutely, or occur repeatedly, to cause chronic inflammation, fibrosis and contraction usually of a lower lobe. The pulmonary damage results as much from chemical injury as from the mixed flora. Antibiotics are traditionally prescribed but the underlying

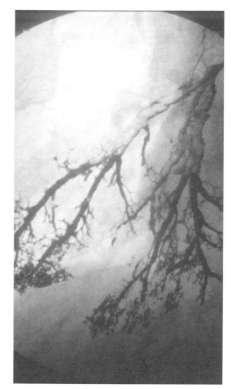

Fig. 3 **Aspiration of barium into lungs in an individual undergoing barium meal examination for swallowing difficulties.**

problem should also be addressed. This may range from anti-reflux manoeuvres to fashioning a tracheostomy.

Case history 9

A 38-year-old previously well woman presented with a left upper and lower lobe pneumonia. Her right lung was clinicoradiologically normal. She was treated with parenteral cefotaxime and a macrolide. High-dose flucloxacillin was added on day 2 when *Staphylococcus aureus* grew in blood and sputum cultures. Four days later she remains unwell with a persistent and swinging fever and persisting pleurisy. Concerns?

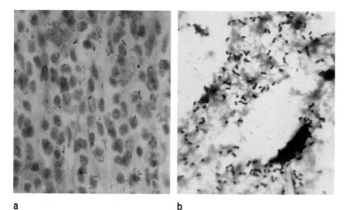

a   b

Fig. 2 **Sputum microscopy. (a)** Mycobacteria. **(b)** *Streptococcus pneumoniae*.

Pneumonia

- There are no clinicoradiological features of pneumonia that allow prediction of the microbiological cause.
- Antibiotic therapy must be started promptly and must cover likely infecting organisms.
- The spectrum of infection in nosocomial pneumonia is very different from community infections, with more Gram-negative bacteria. The initial blind therapy requires antibiotics with a differing spectrum of activity.

MYCOBACTERIAL INFECTIONS I

Mycobacteria are ubiquitous bacilli that include pathogens of man, mammals including cattle and badgers, and reptiles. Since ancient times they have caused human infection as:

- leprosy (caused by *Mycobacterium leprae*), not considered further here
- tuberculosis, both pulmonary and extrapulmonary disease caused by a group of similar mycobacteria termed *Mycobacterium tuberculosis* complex
- more indolent infection caused by a number of environmental opportunistic mycobacteria.

They grow more slowly than conventional bacteria so human infections tend to be chronic and require lengthy treatment.

DETECTION

Microscopy

In the laboratory they can be recognised, once stained, by a characteristic of resisting subsequent decolorisation by both acid and alcohol in a Ziehl-Neelson technique ('acid and alcohol fast bacilli'). Microscopic examinations may be of neat or concentrated specimens such as sputum, pleural fluid or biopsies of pleura or bone marrow. Specimens are 'smear positive' if mycobacteria are present in sufficient concentration to be detected. If this is sputum, the patient is conventionally considered infectious. However, such staining does not discriminate between viable and dead bacteria that may be coughed up after effective therapy for pulmonary disease. Nor does it discriminate between *Mycobacteria tuberculosis* and other pathogenic or environmental mycobacteria that may be present. In much of the world this is the only means of diagnosis.

Culture

Conventional culture on solid Lowenstein–Jensen medium is selective for mycobacterial growth but requires weeks. This delays confirmation of microscopy results, organism identification and antibiotic sensitivities. The latter is invaluable if the mycobacteria are drug-resistant, but otherwise in vitro testing of single antibiotics does not predict the effectiveness of drug combinations in vivo.

Rapid culture techniques have thus been developed which detect either specific metabolism or genetic material.

Molecular techniques

Techniques are available that detect trace amounts of mycobacterial genetic material and even drug resistance. Especial care is necessary in the interpretation of results as contamination by genetic material from environmental non-pathogenic mycobacteria risks false positives. Though not replacing conventional culture, the rapidity of a result within a few hours may be useful in diagnosing infection in immunosuppressed individuals. However, the expense of these techniques means that they are unlikely to become widely available quickly.

The identification of organism-specific, unique genome sequences, 'genetic fingerprinting', has been used in the investigation of outbreaks of tuberculosis. It has provided fascinating information on high rates of re-infection rather than re-activation.

TUBERCULOSIS

Infection by *Mycobacteria tuberculosis* has been with man since ancient times. The first epidemics probably occurred when hunter-gathers began to gather into close communities with cattle. As we enter the third millennium AD, tuberculosis remains a global threat to health. At least one-third of the world's population is now infected and tuberculosis will be responsible for one-quarter of all preventable adult deaths. In developing countries, where more than 90% of the deaths will occur, many patients are economically active adults. Following earlier decades of apathy, the 1990s saw national and international agencies struggling with inadequate resources to control the modern epidemics of tuberculosis and of HIV co-infection.

Prevention and control

Strategies necessary to control tuberculosis in communities were in place in the UK before modern, effective drug therapy became available. The importance of good nutrition, pasteurised milk, tuberculin testing of herds, adequate sanitation and less crowded housing were recognised and variously implemented in the early 1900s. Identifying and removing infectious patients to sanatoria where they received fresh air and good food interrupted transmission. These benefits were illustrated by incidence and death rates falling long before effective chemotherapy became available. Interrupting the cycle of transmission is just as important today (see p. 2).

Vaccination

The intradermal injection of a live attenuated strain of *Mycobacterium bovis*, bacille-Calmette–Guérin (BCG), generates a T_{h1}-cell-mediated immune response in the majority of recipients. This response protects against subsequent intracellular infection by recognising and destroying macrophages laden with mycobacteria.

It is variably effective against mycobacterial infection, particularly for childhood miliary infection and meningitis. It is less effective in some communities, such as eastern Africa, for the more infective forms of tuberculosis. The protection provided by BCG vaccination is not dependent on subsequent skin test reactivity.

The widespread vaccination of young teenagers when the community incidence of tuberculosis was appreciable contributed to falling notification rates in the UK. The current value of BCG vaccination in low incidence communities is less easy to appreciate. Society may need reminding that with readily available and ever cheaper air travel, the epidemics of Africa and Asia are ours too. BCG will provide protection against ordinary and drug-resistant strains of tuberculosis.

Skin testing

The intradermal injection of a purified protein derivative (tuberculin PPD) of *Mycobacterium tuberculosis* stimulates T_{h2}-cell-mediated hypersensitivity. This has a necrotising granulomatous skin response in some individuals with prior immunological experience of mycobacteria, including BCG. It is administered either as a single procedure multiple injection Heaf test (Fig. 1), or as a Mantoux test by a series of single injections with increasing doses of PPD. The skin reaction 3–7 days later is measured as either the pattern of skin response to the multi-injection test or the extent of skin induration to sequential Mantoux injections.

The test is used prior to BCG vaccination to identify patients with immunological experience who would not benefit from further vaccination. Patients with an exaggerated response suggestive of recent infection may also be identified.

The value of skin tests in the diagnosis of tuberculosis is limited. Previous BCG vaccination, the delay between exposure and the development of cutaneous reactivity, and the effect of intercurrent illnesses may all affect the results of correctly administered skin tests.

Case notification

Informing health authorities following the diagnosis of a new patient with tuberculosis is a statutory requirement in several countries. It triggers screening procedures centring on the new 'index' case and provides epidemiological data.

Screening

In recognising person–person transmission as the means of spreading tuberculosis, 'screening' was developed over 100 years ago. It is the proactive seeking of disease arising either as a source for, or spread from, the index case. Screening of whole communities to identify new cases by mass miniature chest radiography continued until the 1960s. It was abandoned when more tumours than tuberculosis were being discovered. Screening is now usually limited to household cases of non-infectious disease, but includes workplace and other casual contacts of infectious cases. Contacts are examined clinically with a skin test and, often, a radiograph.

PRIMARY TUBERCULOSIS INFECTION

Human tuberculosis infection occurs either by inhalation of respirable droplets containing *Mycobacteria tuberculosis* from an infective contact, or by ingestion of milk from tuberculous-infected cows. Inhaled organisms are taken up by alveolar macrophages and initiate an inflammatory response with granuloma formation and enlargement of the local

Grade		Description	
0	to	From nothing to feel to no more than 3 raised spots	Negative: no previous immunological experience
1	to	4 to 6 separate raised spots	Weak reaction: previous environmental mycobacteria infection or weak BCG response
2		6 raised spots forming a circle	Previous infection or BCG response
3		Coalescence with raised centre	Previous event recent, infection, may have been subclinical
4		Blisters	Previous, even recent infection may have been subclinical

a
Fig. 1 **Heaf skin testing (b) and reactions (a) with some of their implications.**

draining lymph nodes (Fig. 2). This response is often effective at containment; only about 10% of individuals infected develop clinical disease. With time the sites of inflammation within the lung and local nodes fibrose and calcify. In the lungs this is called a Gohn focus. The patient's tuberculin skin test will have become positive. If the immunological reaction occurs close to the pleura, a lymphocyte-rich inflammatory pleural effusion develops. A high clinical suspicion is necessary as mycobacteria are scarce on examination of pleural fluid or biopsy.

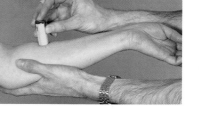

b

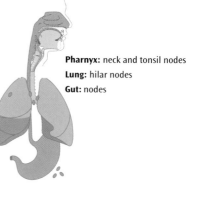

Pharnyx: neck and tonsil nodes
Lung: hilar nodes
Gut: nodes

Fig. 2 **Primary tuberculosis infection.** Inhaled organisms cause a primary response in the respiratory tract. Ingested organisms result in a primary intestinal complex.

Dissemination

If the host's response to this primary infection is inadequate, because of either age or intercurrent disease or treatment, the organisms overwhelm local defences and dissemination occurs with clinical disease and a large burden of mycobacteria. Spread directly via the bronchial tree causes tuberculous bronchopneumonia. More importantly, dissemination via the lymphatics or the bloodstream causes either tuberculous meningitis or miliary tuberculosis. Both can be rapidly lethal and difficult to diagnose clinically.

Case history 10

A 25-year-old Caucasian student travels overland to Australia from western Europe taking 12 months. Once there she seeks help concerning tuberculosis. She has no symptoms or respiratory signs, but does have a BCG scar. A Heaf skin test demonstrates a blistering grade 4 reaction. What does this mean?

Mycobacterial infections I

- Tuberculosis is now a global threat to health due more to social inequalities than to medical issues.
- BCG vaccination provides some protection against mycobacterial infection.
- Tuberculin skin testing is useful in the control of tuberculosis, but is of limited use in the diagnosis, especially in populations that have received prior BCG vaccination.
- Increasingly, new adult cases are being recognised as re-infection rather than as reactivation.

MYCOBACTERIAL INFECTIONS II

POST-PRIMARY TUBERCULOSIS

This is the usual presentation of disease in developed countries. Long after the primary infection, clinically apparent disease of especially lungs, kidneys and bones occurs (Fig. 1). This reactivation of latent mycobacterial dissemination is due to waning immunity with advancing age, intercurrent illnesses, including protein-calorie malnutrition and HIV infection, and intercurrent immunomodulating treatment in developed countries, including steroids. Recent molecular techniques are raising the possibility that at least some clinical cases conventionally considered post-primary reactivation are truly re-infection.

Pulmonary disease usually presents as an upper lobe pneumonia with the radiological development of cavitation and contralateral disease. Malaise, weight loss and cough are prominent, although haemoptysis is not, unless there is associated bronchiectasis. The radiographic abnormalities are often out of proportion to the pulmonary clinical signs detected. Differential diagnoses must include other causes of pneumonia, chronic eosinophilic pneumonia and malignancy. Patients expectorating sputum that is positive on direct microscopic examination for mycobacteria are infectious, responsible for the person–person transmission of disease. They are the most sought-after patients in any disease control programme.

Tuberculous empyema usually develops as an encysted pleural effusion with non-specific systemic upset. The diagnosis is made by pleural biopsy which demonstrates characteristic granulomas, sometimes with organisms visible on direct staining. Pleural biopsy culture is most likely to provide confirmation.

Miliary tuberculosis is an uncommon presentation. However, unlike most other presentations of tuberculosis, diagnosis can be difficult and miliary tuberculosis can be rapidly fatal. There is no pulmonary feel to the presentation, which may be a steady decline with a low-grade fever termed 'cryptic miliary tuberculosis'. A high index of clinical suspicion is needed. Material for culture that may include sputa and bone marrow should be rapidly acquired and adequate drug therapy commenced early, looking for a clinical response before bacterial confirmation. In the UK most patients dying from tuberculosis die with either unrecognised miliary disease or soon

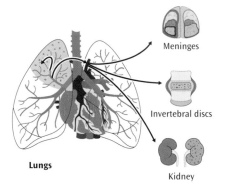

Fig. 1 **Post-primary tuberculosis infection with haematogenous spread.** Infection occurs in many other organ systems, especially bone, brain and urinary tract.

after presentation. Such mortality rates have not fallen over the decades. In developing countries patients die due to progressive disease.

NON-PULMONARY MANIFESTATIONS OF TUBERCULOSIS

Skeletal tuberculosis infection affects the spine more than long bones. Bone destruction occurs without new bone formation, resulting in deformation, pain and instability with potential nerve entrapment (Fig. 2). Adequate drug treatment rapidly relieves pain and usually avoids the need for surgical intervention.

Renal tract tuberculosis. Progressive renal fibrosis with loss of function and later calcification is uncommon. Ureteric strictures will worsen after the commencement of adequate chemotherapy with rapid decline in renal function. This is important to identify and pre-empt with concomitant steroid therapy.

Lymph node tuberculosis usually involves the cervical glands which enlarge and ulcerate.

Neurological involvement may occur as a consequence of skeletal involvement. Tuberculous meningitis is an uncommon but potentially fatal manifestation with coma, fits, cranial nerve and cerebral damage with hydrocephalus.

Gastrointestinal tract tuberculosis, usually of the the terminal ileum, has been abolished in developed communities. In communities where cattle are not tested and live in close contact with humans, gastrointestinal tuberculosis may still be found.

Systemic features of untreated tuberculosis include prominent weight loss and emaciation. Lassitude is common

with adrenal infection and subsequent hypoadrenalism. Skin infection, such as lupus vulgaris, requires differentiation from cutaneous sarcoid.

TREATMENT

The first 80 years of the 20th century saw effective drugs and regimes develop. The last 20 saw the necessity of these strategies demonstrated by the emergence of drug-resistant tuberculosis as a worldwide threat to public health.

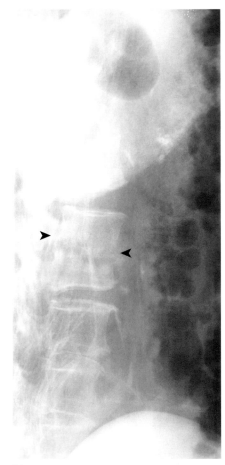

(a)

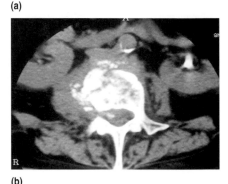

(b)

Fig. 2 **Bone tuberculosis. (a)** Plain radiograph of lumbar vertebral end plate destruction (arrows) by tuberculosis. **(b)** CT of lumbar vertebral body destruction by tuberculosis.

Effective treatment is based on the principles of:

- **Organism sensitivity to drugs.** Primary, naturally-occurring, resistance of mycobacteria occurs infrequently to each individual drug, for example about 1 bacterium in 10^9 are naturally resistant to rifampicin, and 1 in 10^6 to isoniazid. Treatment of clinical disease with either drug will produce an initial clinical response while selecting out for continued growth of the drug-resistant mutant. Later relapse occurs unresponsive to either re-introduction, or continuation, of the initial treatment.

- **Mycobacteria subpopulations.** Most of the infecting mycobacteria are rapidly dividing and readily susceptible to drug therapy. However, small numbers may remain in acidic, hypoxic environments. Still others may be metabolically dormant until they undergo occasional spurts of metabolism rendering themselves vulnerable to drugs. Drug regimes have to be effective against all subpopulations to cure (Fig. 3).

Drug regimes

The fundamental principle is to use at least two drugs to which the organism is fully sensitive at all times. Modern curative, but expensive, short course chemotherapy uses an induction phase of four drugs (rifampicin, isoniazid, pyrazinamide and ethambutol) for 2 months. Rifampicin and isoniazid are then continued for 4 more months.

Other equally effective regimes use drugs, such as para-aminosalicylate or thioacetazone, that are cheaper; however,

the incidence of side-effects is higher and treatment regimes longer. Unfortunately, the availability of the highly effective, but expensive, drug rifampicin is limited in developing countries, where much of the disease burden lies. Thrice weekly intermittent regimes are as effective as daily therapy and may be easier to supervise. Such supervision of drug therapy may be extended to direct observation of drug ingestion to prevent inadequate therapy, particularly premature termination of therapy once patients feel better.

Chemoprophylaxis

Individuals infected with tuberculosis but free of active disease may be treated with short courses of one or two anti-tuberculous drugs. The rationale is that they have a small burden of microbes.

Drug-resistant tuberculosis

Inadequate drug therapy will select mycobacteria resistant to either single or multiple drugs: MDR tuberculosis (Tb). The result is treatment failure with disease relapse. Increasingly, transmission of drug-resistant disease to new hosts is occurring. Outbreaks of resistant disease have occurred in the UK and North America and the incidence is rising. In parts of Asia, 50% of sputum cultures are MDR Tb. Treating patients with MDR Tb is difficult and initially requires five previously unused drugs at adequate dose, patient isolation and strict, directly observed therapy.

Surgery for pulmonary tuberculosis

Before effective drug therapy, surgical techniques were developed with some success to collapse and rest an infected lobe or lung. With drug-resistant tuberculosis there is a revival of techniques to reduce the bacterial load and assist drug action.

Immunotherapy

Use of *M. vaccae* as an adjunct to drug therapy may favourably manipulate the host's immune response away from tissue damage and towards bactericidal action.

CO-INFECTION WITH HUMAN IMMUNODEFICIENCY VIRUS (HIV).

In many parts of the developing world, especially Africa and the Far East, tuberculosis now co-exists with HIV infection. Dual infection increases HIV replication, thus accelerating the decline in immunity. The presence of HIV makes clinical tuberculosis more likely and more aggressive but more likely to be sputum smear negative.

OPPORTUNISTIC MYCOBACTERIA

Individuals infected are not usually immunodeficient but have pre-existing chronic lung disease that provides a niche for bacterial colonisation and subsequent infection. Pulmonary infection is typically slowly progressive and in the upper lobe. There are a number of pathogens with a geographical variation that reflects the environmental burden. *M. xenophi* is a common pathogen in the south of the UK and *M. kansasii* predominates in the Midlands. By contrast, *M. malmoense* is commonest in the cooler north but is more aggressive and can cause progressive pulmonary disease indistinguishable from *M. tuberculosis*. Eradication is more difficult, involving prolonged therapy with ethambutol and rifampicin. Some of the newer macrolide and quinolone antibacterials have useful activity.

Mycobacteria avium-intracellulare (MAI or MAIC) causes serious opportunistic infection in patients suffering from AIDS. Elimination is often not possible and lifetime suppressant therapy is required.

> ### Case history 11
>
> An immigrant arrives by air from an Asian country and undergoes routine health screening. A chest radiograph is abnormal and sputa smear positive for mycobacteria. What needs to be done?

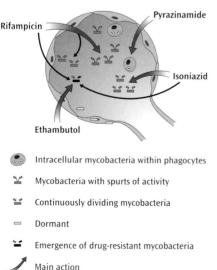

Rifampicin

Pyrazinamide

Isoniazid

Ethambutol

- Intracellular mycobacteria within phagocytes
- Mycobacteria with spurts of activity
- Continuously dividing mycobacteria
- Dormant
- Emergence of drug-resistant mycobacteria
- Main action

Fig. 3 **Tuberculosis subpopulations and drugs.**

> ## Mycobacterial infections II
>
> - Tuberculosis can infect any organ system and so frequently appears as a differential diagnosis.
> - The well established principles of effective disease management must be followed to ensure successful eradication. Drug treatment of tuberculosis requires conscientious taking of combination drug therapy supervised by an appropriately experienced specialist.
> - HIV co-infection and MDR Tb are both increasing and global health issues. In the UK they often co-exist: MDR Tb is more likely in a patient with AIDS.
> - Non-tuberculous mycobacteria require protracted combination drug therapy based on clinical experience rather than in vitro drug sensitivity patterns.

FUNGAL DISEASES

Fungi and their spores are everywhere in the environment. Skin infection is common as a result of the largest interface with the environment but respiratory infections are second in frequency and more common in warmer climates. Pulmonary infection is due to either:

- opportunistic pathogens, or
- endemic pathogens.

OPPORTUNISTIC PATHOGENS

Candida

The organism that causes thrush, *C. albicans*, lives on our bodies with other bacteria. It multiplies and coalesces into pale plaques of clinically apparent infection when either host defences are impaired or the population of resident commensal bacteria are disturbed. Such mechanisms include the use of broad-spectrum antibiotics, oral or inhaled corticosteroids, diabetes mellitus or HIV infection. Although the oropharyngeal mucosa is a common site for *Candida* infection as 'thrush', further extension into the lower respiratory tract is rare. Even in AIDS, where oropharyngeal and oesophageal thrush can be an early and severe feature, endobronchial plaques and *Candida* pneumonia are rare. Septic pulmonary emboli can arise from infected intravascular catheters.

Aspergillus

Aspergillus is a ubiquitous mould that in western Europe liberates its spores into the atmosphere in autumn and winter. It is responsible for the majority of fungal respiratory disease as an opportunistic pathogen. It causes respiratory disease as:

- **Allergic bronchopulmonary aspergillosis (ABPA).** Inhaled *A. fumigatus* spores reside within bronchi and incite an allergic type I immunological reaction with wheeze, breathlessness, cough and a peripheral blood eosinophilia. The scant intrabronchial fungi, together with the host's inflammatory response, especially eosinophils and mucus, form casts of the bronchi which may be coughed up. Fungal fragments with a ragged appearance may be seen in these plugs. They may also obstruct bronchi and cause distal lung infiltration and collapse, usually associated with increased symptoms. However, it may occasionally be asymptomatic and only demonstrable on a chest radiograph. Untreated, the chronic inflammation with localised airway damage and sputum retention results in proximal cystic bronchiectasis. Patients with ABPA should be positively identified from other atopic asthmatics. They characteristically have:
  - a history of expectorating airway casts
  - a peripheral blood eosinophilia when not taking oral steroids
  - an immediate skin weal and flare response to a prick test of an extract of *Aspergillus*
  - variable chest radiographic infiltrates occurring autumn to winter and which may be asymptomatic.

  Such patients require long-term continuous steroid therapy to reduce the resulting lung damage and progression to bronchiectasis. Oral steroids are traditional but high dose inhaled may be an alternative.

- **Mycetoma (aspergilloma).** A ball of fungus develops within a pre-existing lung cavity. Such cavities are usually the result of tuberculosis infection, but may have arisen by other pathology, including lung infarction. Fungal spores, usually *Aspergillus*, are inhaled into the cavity, the fungus grows along the cavity floor and walls eliciting an inflammatory response. When it is extensive, this lining falls in on itself and coalesces together as a mass. This ball then enlarges and the air rim around it produces a

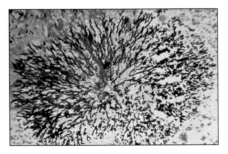

Fig. 2 **Histology of necrotising pulmonary *Aspergillus*.** Reproduced with permission from Bayer plc.

  characteristic crescent on a chest radiograph (Fig. 1). The local inflammatory response is intense and often visible radiographically by the development of marked pleural thickening overlying the cavity. This may be noticed radiographically before the aspergilloma itself is visible. Systemic antibodies are present as *Aspergillus* precipitins. Systemic symptoms are usually slight. Occasionally the fungal ball is coughed out. Sometimes haemoptysis occurs which may be life threatening. When the ball fills the available cavity, further growth causes pressure necrosis of the surrounding cavity wall and lung with haemorrhage. If haemoptysis or systemic upset requires treatment, local or systemic antifungal therapy is less hazardous, but surgical attempts to excise the cavity may be necessary.

- **Extrinsic allergic alveolitis (EAA).** *A. clavatus* thrives in the warm, damp and dark environment of malting kilns where barley is germinated to malt. Following exposure to inadequately ventilated work areas or to mouldy barley elsewhere, workers develop the

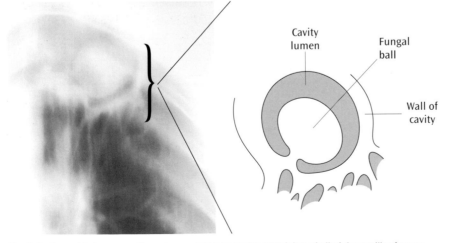

Fig. 1 **Radiographic tomogram through an apical lung cavity containing a ball of *Aspergillus* fungus – an aspergilloma.**

Cavity lumen

Fungal ball

Wall of cavity

features typical of acute EAA: breathlessness, cough, fevers and lung crackles with a radiological lung infiltrate. This form of occupational alveolitis has been termed 'malt worker's lung'.

- **Necrotising pulmonary aspergillosis.** This usually occurs when patients are severely immuno-compromised, such as following solid organ transplantation. Occasionally diabetes mellitus, alcoholism or intercurrent viral infection may be the only risk factors identifiable. The diagnosis can be difficult to make in life. In an appropriate patient the demonstration by tissue biopsy, or distal lung lavage at bronchoscopy, of even one colony of dividing *Aspergillus* is important. Treatment often needs to be started empirically looking for evidence of a clinical response (Fig. 2).

Cryptococcus neoformans
This yeast causes infection in immuno-suppressed patients who have had contact with bird, particularly pigeon, droppings. It may be a cause of acute pneumonia, even of immunocompetent patients in the tropics. It usually causes an acute lymphocytic meningitis, particularly in AIDS patients.

Endemic pathogenic fungi
These often have a characteristic geographical distribution that reflects environmental factors: soil biology or specific microenvironments (Fig. 3). Able to cause disease in previously healthy indi-viduals, they can cause devastating infection in immunocompromised patients.

- **North America:** *Histoplasma* (also Africa), *Blastomyces* (also the Middle East), *Coccidioides*.
- **South America:** *Paracoccidioides, Coccidioides, Histoplasma*.

Histoplasma, Blastomyces, Coccidioides, Paracoccidioides
These dimorphic fungi exist in soil as moulds, but are able to change into patho-genic yeasts at a higher ambient temperature. *Histoplasma* is particularly associated with bird and bat communities and the damp river valleys of eastern America. *Coccidioides* prefers a more arid environment.

When the moulds are disturbed and inhaled into the warmer temperatures of animal and human lungs they become pathogenic yeasts. The inhaled infecting dose is the major determinant of the clinical illness.

A large acute exposure, such as occurs when bird or bat roosting sites are disturbed, is likely to cause a systemic illness with erythema nodosum, musculoskeletal symptoms as well as respiratory distress with bilateral pulmonary infiltrates. Progressive systemic disease is rare following single acute exposures.

Chronic low level exposure causes chronic relapsing malaise, weight loss with systemic manifestations, including pulmonary infiltration and cavitation, not dissimilar to tuberculosis. Chest radio-graphs demonstrate scattered opacities which may calcify.

DIAGNOSIS OF FUNGAL INFECTION
Early diagnosis is not easy. The important step is to think of the possibility of fungal disease. Though many are endemic, the ease of international travel now means that fungal disease can present in non-endemic areas. Enquiring about a patient's travel history is thus crucial.

Biopsy with staining and culture for fungi should be attempted. Biopsy mater-ial, such as of lung, liver and marrow, should be examined with sputum and broncho-alveolar lavage. Culture can be frustratingly slow. A variety of assays for antigen are available and can provide early information. Serology is only useful retrospectively or in chronic disease. Skin tests, though easy, can be misleading.

TREATMENT OF FUNGAL DISEASES
Treatment with parenteral amphotericin is the mainstay of therapy, although allergic, renal and liver toxicity are particularly fre-quent. These effects may be ameliorated by the use of lipid emulsion or liposomal preparations. There is increasing experi-ence in the use of the imidazoles for sys-temic fungal infections. Parenteral ketoconazole for systemic *Candida* infec-tion and oral itraconazole for *Aspergillus* appear useful. Flucytosine is useful in conjunction with amphotericin in crypto-coccal infections. Early diagnosis and prompt antifungal therapy is not always sufficient. The outcome of such treatment is also dependent on the patient and their immunological competence.

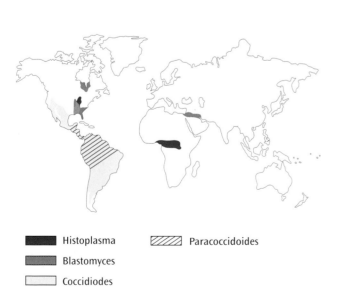

Fig. 3 **Distribution of endemic fungi that cause human pulmonary disease.**

■ Histoplasma   ▨ Paracoccidoides
■ Blastomyces
□ Coccidiodes

Case history 12
An otherwise well 54-year-old woman with diabetes melli-tus is admitted to an intensive care unit in respiratory dis-tress with pneumonia. Early bronchoscopy yields *Staphylococcus aureus* and *Aspergillus* readily on culture. Comment on the significance of the fungal isolate.

Fungal diseases
- Think of fungal infection especially: fever in immunosuppressed patients returning from areas with endemic pathogenic fungi.
- Diagnosis of invasive fungal disease is not easy and therapy may not always be successful.
- *Aspergillus* is the fungus responsible for a range of pulmonary conditions in the UK.

EMPYEMA AND LUNG ABSCESS

EMPYEMA

Empyema (thoracis) describes pus within the pleural space. It can arise either de novo or complicating infection elsewhere, usually pulmonary. With the widespread use of antibiotics, empyemas have become relatively uncommon but may then be overlooked until late.

When complicating pneumonia, an empyema arises as sepsis spreads into a pleural effusion adjacent to the consolidation. Many of these sympathetic effusions are cell-rich. Undoubtedly, a spectrum of pleural fluid appearances exists in relation to pneumonia from straw-coloured transudates through cloudy parapneumonic effusion to frank pus (Fig. 1). Rarely is the spread of infection the direct result of destruction through the visceral pleura. Such destructive infections tend to be due to *Staphylocci* or Gram-negative organisms in a debilitated patient. Occasionally the infection arises as septicaemic spread from a site of infection outwith the thorax, such as the oropharynx.

Many pleural infections are primary infections without an infective source elsewhere. In these cases the commonest infecting organism is *Streptococcus melleri* or *Mycobacteria tuberculosis*.

Clinical features

The features of a primary empyema are fever with systemic upset and pleural discomfort. The empyema may involve the whole pleural space, when there will be signs of pleural fluid on examination (Fig. 2). Encysted infections will produce more localised signs. There may also be evidence of predisposing factors that include diabetes and poor dentition. In all such cases urgent pleural aspiration with a large bore needle able to aspirate viscid material is required to determine the nature of the pleural fluid. Following confirmation of pleural pus, aggressive drainage should be instituted.

When associated with a pneumonia, the presence of any pleural fluid may be less obvious especially in a patient severely ill. Any failure to respond to appropriate antibiotics or lack of resolution of a fever should prompt a clinical and radiographic search for pleural infection. Chest radiography may demonstrate a pleural effusion or the typical D-shaped shadow of encysted pleural fluid (Fig. 3). Pleural ultrasound may then identify the optimal site for aspiration and drainage.

Chronic empyemas may cause prolonged systemic upset with the development of finger clubbing and rarely amyloid.

Management

Turbid parapneumonic effusions should be aggressively drained to dryness via a large bore intercostal tube drain. Straw-coloured fluid in association with a pneumonia should at least be aspirated and if neutrophil-rich or culture positive should be drained. Purulent fluid must also be drained through large bore intercostal tubes with the aim of draining to dryness, sterilising and closing the pleural cavity. Intracavitary fibrinolytic agents such as streptokinase have been used successfully to aid drainage without systemic disturbances in blood coagulation. Radiological assistance may be required to optimally site a drain and occasionally surgical rib resection is required either to gain access to the pleural cavity or to remove gelatinous debris. Antibiotic therapy is a lesser part of management but selection should either be governed by culture results or be broad and include activity against anaerobes.

All patients with an empyema deserve bronchoscopy to exclude underlying lung disease, especially bronchial obstruction by tumour or foreign body.

Thoracic surgery

The exuberant inflammatory pleural thickening that develops around pleural empyemas may fibrose. Unless judiciously removed by surgical 'decortication', this fibrosed thickening will prevent the underlying lung from fully re-expanding and in time will calcify, permanently restricting respiratory move-

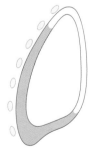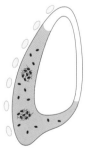

Inflammatory fluid collects in pleura adjacent to pneumonia

Fluid rich in fibrin precursors and cells matrix of fibrin and inflammatory cells
Fluid thickens
Organisms present

Viscid pus with intense inflammatory rind to it

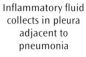

Fig. 1 **The development of an empyema.**

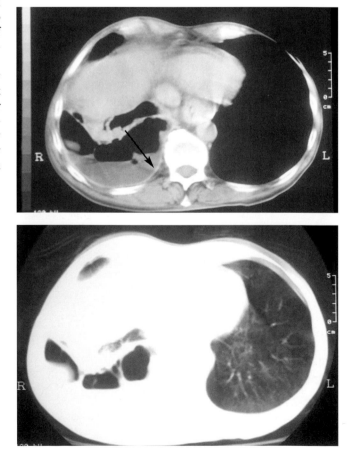

Fig. 2 **CT with pleural enhancement (arrow) and several gas-fluid levels.**

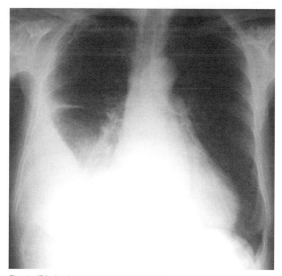

Fig. 3 'D' shadow on chest radiograph.

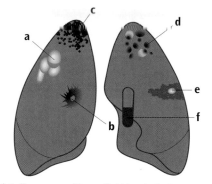

a) Bullae, some with gas-fluid levels that raise the possibility of infection

b) Caviting squamous lung cancer, note thick wall and spiculated periphery

c) Pneumonia with apparent cavities: either true cavitation/necrosis or pneumonia in emphysematous lung.

d) Rheumatoid lung nodes that may cavitate in coal workers (Caplan's syndrome)

e) Peripheral consolidation to a pleural surface of a pulmonary infarct with cavitation

f) Thin, more regular, walled cavity with gas fluid level of a purulent abscess

Fig. 4 Radiographic appearances of lung abscesses and other cavitating lesions.

ments. If there is air within the empyema cavity, helical CT scanning may give pre-operative confirmation of a broncho-pleural fistula which would limit the extent of decortication.

Empyemas occasionally develop in a pneumonectomy space following break-down at the bronchial stump suture line. This is very serious, as the cavity can never be sterilised of infection. Rib resection and long-term tube drainage are required.

LUNG ABSCESS

Intrapulmonary cavities with pus develop occasionally in the context of suppurating pneumonia with lung destruction, especially by *Staphylococci* or *Klebsiella*. Occasionally in comatosed patients aspiration or regurgitation of stomach contents into the lungs through an unprotected airway may occur. Particles may then cause bronchial obstruction. With associated chemical inflammation and infection, lung suppuration and destruction can occur. Infection distal to bronchial obstruction by a carcinoma may also lead to an abscess.

Clinical features

The features are of pulmonary infection with systemic upset, cough and purulent sputum. There may be the additional features of any underlying condition including tumour. With unrecognised infection, clubbing may develop.

Chest radiography is essential. There may be single or multiple cavities, often with associated pulmonary consolidation. The cavities may contain an air–fluid level appearing as a horizontal edge between cavity and contents on an erect radiograph. A single cavity needs to be distinguished from a cavitating squamous carcinoma or a cavitated pulmonary infarct. Both may give rise to systemic upset and finger clubbing. The wall of a tumour cavity tends to be thicker and more irregular than an abscess cavity. Occasionally a pulmonary infarct may cavitate. Multiple cavities require the active confirmation or exclusion of mycobacterial infection.

Management

Bronchoscopy is indicated in all but the most debilitated patient to ensure bronchial patency and to assist in the confirmation or exclusion of tumour or tuberculosis.

Even with effective antibiotic therapy and patent bronchi, there may still be residual scarring.

Case history 13

A 26-year-old male with insulin-dependent diabetes presents with a 2-week history of chills and malaise, chest pain and increasing breathlessness. On examination he was febrile (38°C) with a stony dull hemi-thorax and opaque on a chest radiograph. What would you now do?

ACTINOMYCOSIS

This Gram-positive bacterium is a usual component of mouth flora. With bad oral hygiene in the context of pulmonary aspiration it can cause pleuropulmonary infections with indolent, usually lower lobe, lung abscesses and empyemas. The latter characteristically is associated with bone involvement and chest wall sinuses, and sometimes with the characteristic discharge of yellow sulphur granules. If diagnosed early the infection responds to high-dose penicillin therapy.

Empyema and lung abscess

- The presence of an empyema must be considered in any patient with clinical or radiological evidence of pleural fluid and a fever.
- Early intervention with antibiotics and pleural drainage is required in all cases of pleural empyema though may not prevent surgical intervention.
- Consider tuberculosis.
- Most single cavitating lesions on chest radiographs in the developed world are malignant.

BRONCHIECTASIS/CYSTIC FIBROSIS

BRONCHIECTASIS

This term describes the clinical picture of dilated damaged bronchi with chronic sepsis. Characteristically, regular sputum production is interspersed with recurrent periods of malaise and worsening respiratory symptoms. It is common in developing countries, though now less common in developed countries as a consequence of better child health. It is almost certainly under-recognised: individuals with chronic sputum production are considered to have chronic bronchitis, especially if cigarette smokers!

Pathogenesis

The cardinal requirements for bronchiectasis to develop are both airway obstruction and infection.

Severe pulmonary infection, is a common precursor especially in childhood when the developing lung is particularly susceptible. Such infections include measles, whooping cough or bacterial pneumonia. Plugs of inspissated mucus or peribronchial fibrosis may provide the obstruction necessary for continuing infection to develop into bronchiectasis. Fibrosis is prominent following tuberculosis infection.

Disturbed mucociliary function is common after infection. Primary cilia dysmotility or abnormal mucus are suggested by the co-existence of bronchiectasis with chronic sinusitis. Male infertility suggests primary cilia dysfunction or cystic fibrosis.

A systemic defect in host defence is uncommon. Immunoglobulin deficiency is the commonest, though HIV infection may be a cause.

Rheumatoid arthritis is associated with recurrent infections that may progress via bronchiolitis to bronchiectasis. Haematological malignancies must at least be considered. Benign endobronchial tumours may be the cause of obstruction.

Cystic fibrosis is an inherited disorder considered further below.

Once infection is established behind obstruction, a vicious cycle of continuing infection, inflammation and local damage is set up. The bacteria involved are not especially virulent but they persist by circumventing host attempts to remove or neutralise them. Products may be released that inhibit ciliary action or mucus function. Paradoxically, much of the lung damage in bronchiectasis is as a result of the host's own inflammatory reaction, especially neutrophils and their toxic products. (Figs 1 & 2).

Clinical

Most patients have a regular cough productive of purulent sputum. This is interspersed with exacerbations when the host–bacteria balance favours bacteria. Systemic upset occurs with fevers, breathlessness and pleurisy, with increased sputum volume and purulence sometimes streaked with blood. Airways obstruction is often present and wheeze may be prominent in a patient's history. A previous severe pulmonary infection may be remembered. Clinical examination demonstrates persistent localised inspiratory crackles on auscultation and often finger clubbing.

Radiology

Plain radiographs are poor for demonstrating bronchiectasis. Round bronchial shadows with air–fluid levels, or the parallel tram-lines of side-on thickened bronchial walls, may be visible. Additional detail can be obtained by high resolution CT lung scanning. Though not indicated in every case, it can confirm the working diagnosis when a chest radiograph is non-contributory. It certainly demonstrates disease extent. CT scanning has now replaced bronchography as the diagnostic gold standard. When bronchiectasis is limited to one lobe only, surgical resection becomes a therapeutic option.

Therapy

Sputum culture will identify colonisation with *Staphylococcus*, *Haemophilus* and probably *Pseudomonas* species. Even fungi and mycobacteria may be present. Continuous antibiotic therapy is of no benefit in suppressing infective exacerbations or preventing colonisation. Indeed it may encourage the development of bacteria resistant to antibiotics. By contrast, antibiotic therapy with appropriate drugs at the time of a clinical exacerbation suppresses bacterial numbers and improves clinical well-being. However, these drugs need to be given at high dose to penetrate the abnormal bronchi into the pus, and for a protracted period. The choice of antibiotic is guided by cultured pathogens and their sensitivity patterns.

Chronic care requires adequate daily physiotherapy. Effective sputum clearance with techniques that include chest percussion and postural drainage are effective in maintaining, if not restoring, some lung function, in reducing exacerbations and preserving quality of life. Airway inflammation should be suppressed with inhaled steroids. There may be associated airflow limitation, even variability, due to bronchial wall inflammation indicating a need for bronchodilator therapy. Disease progression leads to hypoxaemia and respiratory failure. In contrast to patients with cystic fibrosis, patients with other causes of bronchiectasis tend to be treated less aggressively, which may not be appropriate.

It is important to consider underlying causes. Immunoglobulin deficiency can be supported with intravenous globulin products. Localised post-infective bronchiectasis may be amenable to surgical resection. Though mild forms of cystic fibrosis may benefit from gene, or other novel drug, therapy in the future, there are implications for initiating family counselling and screening now.

CYSTIC FIBROSIS

Cystic fibrosis (CF) is the commonest fatal

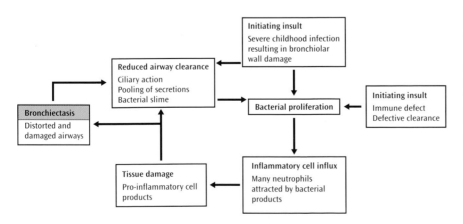

Fig. 1 **Bronchiectasis—the inflammatory vicious circle.**

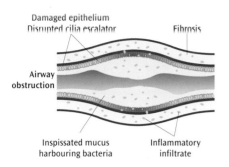

Fig. 2 **Pathology of bronchiectatic airway.**

gene disorder of Caucasians, inherited as an autosomal recessive and with a gene frequency of about 1:25 in at-risk populations. It represents about 1 in 3000–7000 Caucasian births compared to 1:25 000 of Asian descent. The discovery of the CF gene was followed by the characterisation of its defective product. Subsequent interest has focused on the potential for developing novel gene-based therapies.

Clinical features

There is a wide spectrum of clinical severity in this multi-system disease (Fig. 3). The diagnosis should be suspected in any clinical situation that involves more than one system, especially with lung suppuration or pancreatic insufficiency. New diagnoses in adult life are now not infrequent with genotype testing.

The pulmonary consequences of cystic fibrosis represents the severe end of the spectrum of bronchiectasis. Chronic suppurative lung disease usually starts from childhood, progresses to widespread cystic bronchiectasis and is universally present in adult patients. Airways become irreversibly colonised by bacteria. *Pseudomonas* and related species are especially pathogenic, developing into non-mucoid forms that are more resistant to host defences. The presence of *Pseudomonas aeruginosa* and of *Burkolderia cepacia* are separate milestones in the pulmonary decline. Pneumothoraces and haemoptysis that may be life-threatening are frequent respiratory complications. Co-existing chronic sinusitis and nasal polyps are frequent.

Pancreatic glandular secretion fails and bowel obstruction is a presenting feature. Insulin insufficiency is frequent later. Chronic liver disease may develop with portal hypertension and occasionally varices. Male infertility is universal. Malnutrition is multifactorial and impaired growth was frequent in the past.

Treatment

Treatment is multi-system and patient management multi-professional. Chest physiotherapy is the most important aspect of daily care. Inhaled bronchodilators and inhaled steroids may be required and novel anti-inflammatory agents to ameliorate the host's response are being tested. Effective pancreatic enzyme replacement has improved nutrition in successive cohorts of patients. The centralisation of care for patients in special CF units has contributed to the improved survival now seen in many countries. Survival into the third decade is now common, but cardiopulmonary and septic events are often terminal. Heart–lung transplantation can be very successful, but widespread use is limited by donor organ availability.

Genetic aspects

The CF gene was identified in 1989. It is a 250 kilobase gene on the long arm of chromosome 7 coding for a 1480 amino acid structure, the CF transmembrane regulator (CFTR), which appears to be a chloride ion channel. Cellular message was then demonstrated in all tissues affected by the disease clinically and quantitatively similar in both patients and normal individuals. This suggested that the disease was due to subtle molecular abnormalities. Indeed in 70% of CF patients a single amino acid, phenylalanine, has been lost from just one position (the ΔF508 mutation).

Defective CFTR function results in the inability to actively reabsorb chloride from the airway. For reasons not completely understood sodium reabsorption is also increased. Hence the cells' surface becomes more negative in the electrical charge and dehydrated. Coupled with disturbed surface ions, ciliary function is impaired and bacterial adherence may be increased. In the skin, sweat glands behave differently with the sodium passively following the chloride out onto the surface. This abnormal sweat sodium is an important clinical diagnostic test.

Clinical and genetic interactions

Over 300 mutations have been recognised, but intriguingly there appears to be no relation to clinical disease severity.

Prenatal screening for many of the identified CF genotypes is now possible. Antenatal counselling and screening for high-risk couples is available but there are few population-based primary screening programmes yet in place.

Attempts are currently in progress to deliver CFTR gene or message into the airway cells as novel therapy. Even introducing it into nasal epithelium, by either adenovirus or liposomes as vectors, is proving a challenge. Developing drugs to manipulate the function of other airway ion channels to bypass the effects of defective CFTR may be more achievable.

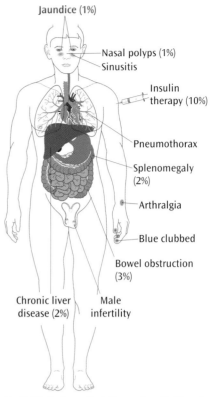

Fig. 3 **Clinical manifestations of cystic fibrosis.** Percentages refer to prevalence at age 20 years.

Case history 14

A 36-year-old, petite, non-smoking women presents with an exacerbation of her 'bronchitis'. She has chronic nasal catarrh and is under investigation for infertility. How would you proceed?

Bronchiectasis/cystic fibrosis

- Bronchiectasis develops as a result of a combination of obstruction and infection. Much resulting lung damage is caused by the host's response to bacterial carriage.
- Chronic sputum production, persistent crackles and finger clubbing suggest the diagnosis. High resolution CT scanning may be needed for confirmation.
- Cystic fibrosis is a lethal recessive genetic disorder of Caucasians. Though over 300 mutations are known (ΔF508 the commonest) there appears to be no good correlation between genotype and clinical picture.
- There is a wide range of clinical expressions of CF in adults, ranging from severe bronchiectasis and respiratory failure to newly diagnosed recurrent bronchitis.

PULMONARY INFECTIONS IN THE IMMUNOCOMPROMISED HOST

Introduction

Patients with impaired immunity are more likely to suffer infective episodes from conventional pathogens as well as clinically important infections caused by organisms that are not usually pathogenic. This latter range of pathogens is large, and has some variation between groups of patients with different causes for immunosuppression. The greatest dichotomy is between patients suffering from AIDS and those with other causes of immunosuppression. For this reason these two patient groups are considered separately.

CAUSES OF COMPROMISED IMMUNOLOGICAL FUNCTION

The disease itself

This involves specific disturbances, such as splenectomy or congenital immunodeficiency syndromes, and more global disorders such as burns, cancer and malnutrition. Haematological malignancies and their treatments produce a profound and chronic immune disturbance.

Immunosuppressing therapy

Therapy comprises corticosteroids, cyclosporin and low-dose chemotherapy, such as cyclophosphamide or azathioprine, following solid organ transplantation and, increasingly, as treatment for immune-mediated diseases. Anti-cancer chemotherapy produces a predictable post-therapy leucopenia and risk of infection. Granulocyte colony-stimulating factors (CSFs) can be used to hasten white cell maturation and release from the bone marrow in conjunction with antibiotics when life-threatening infection is present.

Immunosuppressing infections

The commonest is human immunodeficiency virus (HIV) that causes the acquired immune deficiency syndrome (AIDS). Globally, congenital rubella and the immune paresis immediately following measles infection are important.

PULMONARY INVOLVEMENT

Managing an immunocompromised patient who may have a pulmonary infection is a challenge, not least because they may rapidly deteriorate with overwhelming infection requiring prompt life-saving treatment.

Pulmonary infections usually present with a range of respiratory symptoms, including cough, breathlessness and fever. Sometimes even in the immunocompetent individual there is a complete absence of respiratory symptoms or fever. Sweats and other systemic symptoms may be prominent or relate to the underlying disease. The time course may be rapid with devastating deterioration. Symptoms may also grumble over weeks.

There may be tachypnoea with crackles on chest examination. Lobar consolidation with bronchial breathing should not be expected if there is leucopenia or disturbed leucocyte function since pus will not be formed. The degree of oxygenation must be measured non-invasively by pulse oximetry. Some patients may have unexpectedly profound hypoxaemia which can be diagnostically helpful.

Just as for pneumonia in immunologically competent hosts, there are no clinico-radiological appearances that are unique for selected pathogens. However, a series of chest radiographs can give a time course for the development of pulmonary changes. Detailed CT examinations are often unhelpful but they can localise patchy abnormalities for subsequent invasive sampling.

THE CHALLENGES OF PNEUMONITIS

As well as a range of potentially infectious agents, there may be other causes of similar pulmonary symptoms, signs and radiographic pulmonary infiltrates in these patients.

Underlying disease

- Pulmonary infiltration by leukaemia or lymphoma and lymphangitic spread of malignancy.
- Pulmonary haemorrhage due to thrombocytopenia, either as a direct result of the bone marrow involvement by malignancy or as a result of anti-cancer treatment.

Direct toxic effects of treatment

- Cytotoxic drug therapy may cause predictable pulmonary damage due to a cumulative dose of nitroso-ureas, or may be less predictable with the use of bleomycin or cyclophosphamide. All cause a potentially reversible cellular pneumonitis, but with continuing drug exposure progression to irreversible fibrosis occurs.
- Post-radiotherapy pneumonitis and fibrosis may occur months after high radiation doses. Radiologically, the abnormality reflects the radiotherapy field treated, exhibiting crisp edges and typically abutting the mediastinum. Bleomycin renders the lung radiosensitive, exacerbating radiation damage.

Indirect toxic effects

- Anthracycline chemotherapy agents such as adriamycin may cause a cardiomyopathy. Subsequent pulmonary oedema may develop following apparently trivial fluid challenge and with less than typical radiological appearances.

Miscellaneous causes

- Pulmonary emboli.
- Non-specific pulmonary infiltrates occur following bone marrow transplantation.

INVESTIGATIONS

Lung infections need specific anti-infective therapy if possible and may require

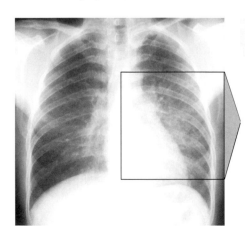

Fig. 1 **Radiograph with abnormalities of a febrile breathless patient on long-term steroid therapy.**

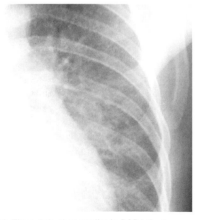

Fig. 2 **The subtle abnormality in PCP infection.**

Table 1 Likely infections in immunodeficiency

Immunodeficiency		Typical clinical scenario
With neutropenia	Without neutropenia	
Gram-negative	Streptococcus	Rapidly progressive
Gram-positive	Haemophilus	Shock
Aspergillus	Legionella	Diffuse lung injury
	Fungi	Moderate progression
	Mycobacteria	Nodular/focal

reduction in the immunosuppressive treatment. By contrast, non-infectious lung involvement by the underlying disease may require increased immunosuppression. Aggressive microbiological investigations, including for fungi, are required.

If sputum is not readily available, induced sputum can be sought by chest physiotherapy following nebulised hypertonic 1.8% saline. Bronchial and pulmonary samples are most useful, though obtainable with varying degrees of difficulty. Many of these patients have a coagulopathy or hypoxaemia complicating their illness which limits bronchoscopy and prevents percutaneous needle biopsy. If mechanical ventilation is likely or helpful then surgical lung biopsy should be considered. All such samples should be examined histologically using stains for the full range of pathogens but also cultured for bacteria, mycobacteria, fungi, viruses and pneumocystis.

If examination of easily obtained samples is unhelpful, a more invasive examination must be individually considered for each patient. Even an open lung biopsy does not always demonstrate the cause of a pulmonary infiltrate or may identify a pathology which has no therapeutic benefit for the patient, such as relapsing acute myeloid leukaemia infiltrating the lung. Conversely, lung biopsy may identify unsuspected pulmonary pathogens or non-infective causes, such as a drug reaction, with significant therapeutic gain. The relatively straightforward technique of thoracoscopic lung biopsy is ideal if available. Patients who are deteriorating fast, with focal rather than diffuse pulmonary abnormalities, recent transplantation, travel or chronic steroid therapy should be biopsied as soon as possible.

PULMONARY INFECTION IN THE HIV-POSITIVE PATIENT

HIV infection impairs immunity by the slow, steady attrition in $CD4^+$ T_h lymphocyte numbers. Moreover, those remaining are impaired in their co-operative interactions with other immune effector cells, including circulating monocytes, macrophages and immunoglobulin-producing B-lymphocytes.

These patients experience a 4-fold increased risk of conventional bacterial pneumonia which tends to be more fulminant. Although patients respond to the usual therapies, relapse is common confirming important interactions between exogenous

antimicrobials and endogenous host defence. Mycobacterial infection with either M. tuberculosis or MAIC occurs especially in areas where tuberculosis is endemic. Fungal infections are uncommon, excepting oropharyngeal thrush. Though cytomegalovirus is commonly isolated from bronchial samples, it rarely causes a pneumonitis.

Pneumocystis carinii

Though the commonest pulmonary infection in these patients, Pneumocystis carinii pneumonia (PCP) can occur in other patients who are chronically immunosuppressed, such as transplant recipients. It is still the AIDS-defining illness in 15% of HIV-infected patients. PCP becomes inevitable when CD4– lymphocyte counts fall below 200 mm^3. This has become the threshold for chemoprophylaxis which has reduced incidence rates, though compliance and drug side-effects remain problems.

Diagnosis of PCP can be difficult. A non-productive cough and progressive breathlessness over several weeks are common symptoms. There may be crackles or the odd wheeze on chest examination, though it is often remarkably normal. Unexpectedly profound arterial hypoxaemia at rest, or particularly upon exercise, is diagnostically useful. Radiological changes can range from bilateral midzone infiltrates to pneumatocele formation to normal appearances, even on high resolution CT scanning. Induced sputum, bronchoscopic lavage or lung biopsy stained with either a silver or fluorescent antibody stain are good means to attempt identification of the pathogen.

Treatment is with high-dose co-trimoxazole, or other antifolate antibiotics, and both corticosteroids that improve survival and appropriate respiratory support. Failure to respond should raise the suspicions of poor compliance or an additional pathogen. Respiratory failure developing in the context of acute PCP has a high mortality.

PULMONARY INFECTION IN THE IMMUNOCOMPROMISED NON-HIV-POSITIVE PATIENT

Though there is a wide range of potential pathogens, the principles of history and examination and review of all treatments and investigation results, including radiology, are important. The cause of the immunosuppression may give a clue. Conventional nosocomial pneumonia is relatively common in the first few weeks following solid organ transplant, and after 6–12 months, conventional community-acquired pneumonia becomes relatively common. A travel history is important. In patients who have received recurrent courses of broad-spectrum antibiotics consider fungal infection particularly if fungi have been isolated from urine and line sites. In this respect even a single colony of Aspergillus isolated in sputum culture is significant.

Case history 15

A young man presents with 2–3 weeks of increasing breathlessness and a non-productive cough. He looks cyanosed at rest and a few crackles are audible on chest examination. A chest radiograph demonstrates a predominantly unilateral infiltrate. How would you now proceed?

Pulmonary infections in the immunocompromised host

- There are many causes of respiratory illness in immunosuppressed patients, due either to infection, or to underlying disease or its treatment. Elucidation of these causes requires careful consideration of appropriate investigations. All may not be possible or appropriate.

- Pulmonary infections, especially tuberculosis or Pneumocystis carinii may be the presentation of, as well as a complication of, AIDS.

ASBESTOS AND THORACIC DISEASE

ASBESTOS

These naturally occuring mineral fibres are mined for their inert, insulating and fire retardant qualities which has resulted in their widespread use throughout industry. 'Blue' crocidolite asbestos is particularly potent in causing mesotheliomas. The other fibre types, amosite and tremolite, are less potent and the 'white' chrysotile used mainly for building and domestic use appears to be the least harmful. Types of employment where asbestos exposure has occurred in the past include:

- ship building and ship breaking yards
- power station building
- marine, naval and heating engineering
- construction work
- packing asbestos as filters for gas masks.

Even exposure received living downwind from a factory, playing with factory waste or as household contact to dust brought home on workers' clothes is risk enough.

INHALATION AND LUNG BEHAVIOUR

Structurally, asbestos fibres are either serpiginous (such as chrysotile) or long, thin and stiff (as are amphiboles including crocidolite and amosite asbestos). These characteristics affect their behaviour within the lungs.

When inhaled, chrysotile penetrates poorly into the lungs, deposits easily and is removed by the mucociliary escalator. Chemically it is less robust and does not seem to last long within the lungs. It has been considered less noxious.

Inhaled amphibole fibres behave as if they were javelins. They penetrate well into the lung peripheries, and probably also into the lung parenchyma. These sharp fibres are less well cleared or engulfed by macrophages, and are chemically more robust. Their movement within the lung is unclear. A few may penetrate directly or be carried by lymph to the pleural surfaces. Subsequently, fibrogenesis or carcinogenesis may occur. The lung attempts to isolate many in an iron–protein coat to become 'asbestos bodies'. These can be identified histologically.

PLEURAL DISEASE

Pleural disease follows the inhaled asbestos fibres either passing via the lymphatics or penetrating directly across the pleural space.

Acute benign pleurisy may occur relatively early after asbestos exposure commences and is often accompanied by an inflammatory and often blood-stained pleural effusion. Though the fluid may recur, spontaneous resolution to pleural thickening is usual.

Parietal pleural plaques of hyaline fibrosis occur increasingly with duration of exposure, especially to the lance-like amphibole asbestos fibres. They are usually bilateral and visible en-face over the mid-lung zones or edge on over the diaphragm surfaces. They may calcify over time, are clinically silent and are not pre-malignant (Fig. 1).

Diffuse pleural thickening may occur extensively over the middle and lower zones of the lung and is also related to accumulative asbestos exposure. In contrast to plaques, diffuse thickening causes breathlessness by restricting thoracic movement.

PARENCHYMAL: FIBROSIS

Asbestosis

This is slowly progressive basal fibrosis following substantial chronic exposure to respirable asbestos fibres. It can be difficult to distinguish from idiopathic pulmonary fibrosis. Other pleuropulmonary evidence of past exposure may be present and progression is slower than idiopathic pulmonary fibrosis. Like any cause of lung fibrosis there is an increased risk of pulmonary malignancies.

AIRWAY DISEASE

Individuals with evidence of asbestos exposure as pleural plaques on chest radiographs may demonstrate evidence of airflow limitation, even if they have not ever smoked. Inhaled asbestos fibre dust causes chronic airway inflammation and airflow limitation.

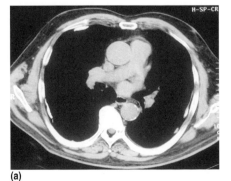

(a)
Fig. 1 **Pleural thickening and calcification of pleural plaques.** Shown on a thoracic CT image slice **(a)** and on X-ray **(b)**.

MALIGNANCY

Lung cancer

Asbestos exposure increases the risk of developing lung cancer and these effects appear to be synergistic with tobacco smoke. There is debate as to whether just heavy exposure to asbestos per se is enough to increase the risk of lung cancer or whether lung fibrosis (asbestosis) is required as a precursor of cancer and therefore an obligate associate.

OTHER MALIGNANCIES

There is some epidemiological evidence to suggest that workers with asbestos exposure have a higher incidence of gastrointestinal and laryngeal cancers. The association is by no means robust nor widely accepted, but in terms of an effect from inhaled or ingested fibres, remains plausible.

Mesothelioma

Mesothelioma is a primary tumour of mesothelial cells of the pleura, occasionally the peritoneum and rarely the pericardium. It represents about 2% of all primary pulmonary malignancies. The majority arise as a consequence of exposure to asbestos fibres, several decades earlier. The risk of pleural mesothelioma does appear to be directly related to both the duration and heaviness of exposure. It is commonly a disease of males aged 50–70 years, with at least 1000 deaths per year in the UK.

Exposure

There is a background incidence of mesothelioma not associated with overt industrial exposures. One of the highest such incidences is in Cappadocia in eastern Turkey, where young adults present

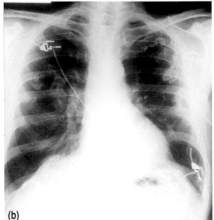

(b)

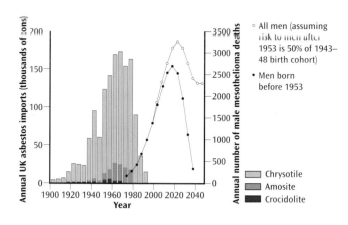

Fig. 2 **Predicted mesothelioma deaths in British men and UK asbestos imports.** (Figure reproduced with permission from Peto Hodgson Matthews and Jones 1995 Continuing increase in mesothelioma mortality in Britain. Lancet 345: 537.)

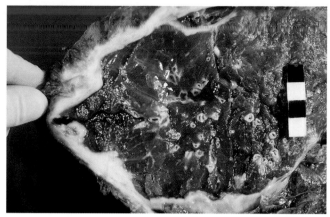

Fig. 3 **Resected lung specimen of mesothelioma illustrating the white tumour spreading along pleural surfaces.**

with this tumour as a result of tremolite, an asbestos-like fibre in the background rock and common in airborne dusts and soil.

As a result of increasing industrial utilisation of asbestos well into the second half of the last century and the time interval between exposure and malignancy, incidence and mortality rates for pleural mesothelioma have steadily risen (Fig. 2). The epidemiological link between asbestos exposure and mesothelioma was made in the middle of the 1960s. Regulations restricting the use of asbestos came into force in the UK in 1969 but were applied variably in the early years. Asbestos has been steadily replaced in many industrial processes by other mineral fibres. Nevertheless, there is an inexorable rise in the incidence of pleural mesothelioma, in part due to incomplete enforcement of the restrictions in the early days and possible carcinogenic potential of the alternative fibres now utilised. Incidence rates are now expected to triple in the next 20 years, and account for more than 1% of male deaths of those born in the 1940s.

Pathology

Mesothelioma may start as a small focus in the pleura with an exuberant pleural effusion. With time the fluid lessens and loculates as the tumour extends along the pleural surface, between lobes and into the lung septae (Fig. 3). Ensnaring the hilar structures results in further loss of lung volume and function. Haematogenous and direct spread into pericardium and across the diaphragm occur late. Most patients will undergo pleural investigation which will demonstrate bloody fluid, with pleural biopsies obtained either by blind percutaneous needle biopsy or under direct vision at thoracoscopy. Interpretation of the histology is not always easy, particularly distinguishing a florid mesothelial reac-

tion from a malignant mesothelioma or metastatic adenocarcinoma. There has always been a concern of tumour spread along the needle track, though this may be rarer than generally thought. Most patients and their doctors are keen for histological confirmation, and any subsequent symptomatic spread can be controlled by local radiotherapy.

Clinical presentation and management

Presentation is typically with either progressive breathlessness or visceral chest pain. Chest examination will demonstrate pleural fluid, confirmed by chest radiology which may demonstrate other features of asbestos exposure. The outlook is poor; median survival from diagnosis is 12–18 months. Though some tumours seem to progress slowly, presentation diagnosis and death inside 6 months is not unheard of. The primary tumour is not radiosensitive and modern chemotherapy regimes have had little impact. If diagnosed early with limited disease, radical surgery as pleuropneumonectomy is possible but with as yet no objective evidence of outcome. The relentless breathless and chest wall pain require proactive anticipation to palliate.

It is a proscribed industrial disease. Patients or their relatives can claim industrial injury disablement benefit, currently £100 per week (2000) tax free. Initiating a civil claim against past employers should be considered, even if the company is no longer trading. Specialist solicitors should be employed and the process is much easier if there is a single employer to pursue in contrast to a number of subcontractors. Even so, such proceedings can be time consuming, costly and with no certainty of a satisfactory outcome. Upon death, the local coroner or procurator fiscal should be notified and an autopsy may be required.

Case history 16

A joiner and a long-standing smoker presents with progressive breathlessness. There are persistent inspiratory crackles to hear over his lung bases and spirometry demonstrates airways obstruction. Opinion?

Asbestos and thoracic disease

- Asbestos exposure causes a range of thoracic abnormalities ranging from benign pleural plaques to malignant mesothelioma.
- Plaques are neither malignant nor pre-malignant and rarely cause symptoms.
- Benign asbestos pleurisy is a diagnosis of exclusion: not all asbestos-related bloody effusions are malignant.
- Mesothelioma can arise following relatively trivial asbestos exposure.
- Pleural mesothelioma is a rare form of cancer, but with a high incidence in areas and occupations where crocidolite blue asbestos has been used.
- Incidence rates are expected to continue to rise into this century. There is current concern about the alternative mineral fibres and the effectiveness of asbestos restrictions.
- Treatment other than symptom palliation has no proven benefit in mesothelioma.

OCCUPATIONAL LUNG DISEASE

Lung disease caused or aggravated by the complex environments of the modern workplace (Fig. 1) is second in frequency only to occupational dermatitis. Knowledge of a patient's current job title alone is insufficient for diagnosis. Specific details of their workplace, the dusts and fumes present and materials used are required. Previous jobs must also be explored chronologically and in detail. Hobbies may be just as relevant too. Errors can be made in both ascribing an occupational cause to a lung condition and failing to appreciate an occupational precipitant. Prevention rather than subsequent treatment of occupational health problems makes medical as well as commercial sense.

In general, single large exposures produce respiratory effects rapidly whereas repetitive low level exposures cause respiratory disease that may be more insidious in onset and progression. The following outlines clinical effects with examples.

UPPER RESPIRATORY TRACT

Acute injury

Direct chemical and thermal injury results in inflammation, necrosis and sloughing of the upper airway mucosa. Chemical injury is more likely to be associated with similar lower respiratory tract effects. There is a real risk of acute airway obstruction. Survival is usually associated with healing but airway support including tracheostomy and mechanical ventilation may be required in the interim. The constituents of domestic house fire smoke include carbon monoxide and cyanides; these are absorbed and block systemic cellular metabolism.

Allergic rhinitis

A blocked stuffy nose or sneezing is often present with occupational asthma or allergic conjunctivitis.

Non-specific irritation

Non-specific irritation by many dusts and chemicals is commonplace. The constellation of symptoms that include cough, dry or runny eyes and nose, headaches and lethargy comprise the 'sick building syndrome'. This results from a dry air-conditioned working environment where employees have inadequate control, perhaps with microbiological contamination.

AIRWAY DISEASE

Occupational asthma

Asthma may be precipitated or worsened by inhalation of work place materials, so a high degree of suspicion and objective evidence are required. Worsening asthma symptoms as a working period progresses with improvement while on holiday or non-working weekends is typical. Confirmation requires PEFR recordings taken each day, ideally 2 hourly, for a whole working week supported with recordings from a weekend or holiday away from work on constant medication (Fig. 2). Occasionally, inhalational exposure challenge testing or a visit to the place of work may be needed.

Industrial processes with volatile organic chemicals, or workers handling natural materials in enclosed environments are usual. The range of at-risk occupations is large and includes acrylic paint-spraying (isocyanates), soldering (colophony flux), bakery (flour), wood working (some timbers), laboratory technicians (animal dander and excreta) and healthcare personnel (latex powder, gluteraldehyde). It is more difficult to

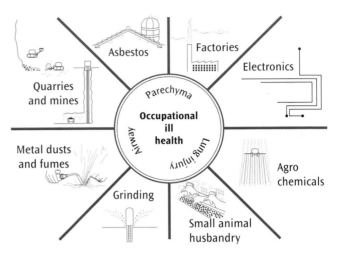

Fig. 1 **Workplace conditions contributing to lung disease.**

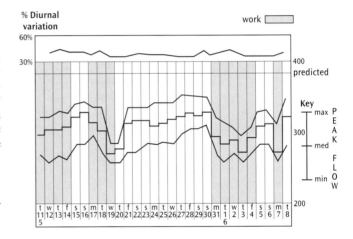

Fig. 2 **Occupational asthma.** Plot of frequently measured peak flow recordings showing deterioration in relation to work and improvement away from the workplace at weekends and during a holiday. This is therefore supportive of occupational asthma. The patient worked in an electronics factory as a solderer.

diagnose when asthma develops in the context of exposures to new chemicals or processes, or where the exposure to recognised allergens is not clear.

Once occupational asthma is diagnosed, effective removal of the chemicals or protection of the worker is required in addition to standard asthma care. In practical terms many workers are unable to change jobs and respiratory protection can be cumbersome. Compensation in the form of industrial injuries benefit may be payable but rarely completely recompenses for loss of earnings. Unfortunately, clinically severe asthma may sometimes persist even following effective worker protection or removal of the chemical.

Identification of occupational asthma also allows protective measures to be introduced to protect other workers.

Byssinosis

This is probably a variation of extrinsic occupational asthma. Workers in the cotton and flax industries develop cough and reversible breathlessness with airways obstruction on exposure to textile fibres and husks contaminated with bacterial and fungal proteins. The clinical features are typically worse at the beginning of a working week. Long-term exposure may result in progressive irreversible airflow limitation.

Reactive airway dysfunction syndrome (RADS)

This is a new term that describes persistent asthma-like airway symptoms that include cough, wheeze and breathlessness developing acutely following a single substantial exposure to an inhaled dust.

Obliterative bronchiolitis

This may occur as a sequel to toxic inhalation with worsening breathlessness and progressive airways obliteration over weeks to months. Gas trapping becomes evident, clinically and radiologically. Nitrogen oxides, especially nitrogen dioxide from agricultural silage or the use of nitro-cellulose explosives in confined spaces, can cause an acute toxic pulmonary oedema which may chronically progress to small airway obliteration.

Chronic bronchitis

Non-specific irritation by inhaled material including cigarette smoke, coal and other dusts causes a chronic productive cough.

Occupational COPD

Increasing recognition of industrial dust and fume exposures that, in addition to cigarette smoke, causes chronic and largely irreversible airways obstruction has prompted the creation of this diagnostic category (Table 1).

PREDOMINANTLY PARENCHYMAL EFFECTS

Toxic

Non-cardiogenic pulmonary oedema can result from inhalation of toxic gases, including chlorine and oxides of nitrogen. These directly cause loss of alveolar–capillary integrity with airspace flooding. Management is supportive and may include mechanical ventilation.

Extrinsic allergic alveolitis (EAA)

This is an immunological interaction occurring in the small airways and lung parenchyma following inhalation of certain organic materials. Acute exposure produces a systemic upset with breathlessness and fever, crackles on auscultation and restriction on pulmonary function testing. Some acute exposures are well recognised, including fungal spores in damp overwintering hay (farmer's lung) or after cleaning pigeon lofts (pigeon fancier's lung). The picture is often confused with infection, and a high index of suspicion is required with a history of appropriate exposure which may be supported by the presence of circulating antibodies. Further exposure is prevented by barrier methods including respirators and modification of the work process or hobby to avoid further exposures.

Repeated or sustained exposure results in progressive breathlessness with lung fibrosis. This may be difficult to confirm clinically and the diagnosis is often supported by high resolution CT lung scanning or lung biopsy. An example is 'budgerigar fancier's lung' where the source of the inhaled feather bloom and avian protein excreta remains in the corner of a patient's room and the progressive breathlessness is erroneously attributed to bronchitis or heart failure.

FIBROSIS

Pneumoconiosis

Over many years of respirable dust exposure, dust-ladened macrophages gather to produce macroscopically visible but asymptomatic deposits a few millimetres in size within the lungs. These produce nodularity on chest radiographs (Fig. 3). Though attributed to inhaling carbonaceous materials, typically coal dust, it is a response to co-existing quartz or other silica in either the native rock or subsequent industrial processes. Simple pneumoconiosis has no clinical consequences unless progressive massive fibrosis develops. This refers to the development of foci of extensive fibrosis usually in the upper lung zones that can develop after dust exposure has ceased. Though it may cause exertional breathlessness and cough it is usually a radiographic diagnosis.

Silicosis

Respirable crystalline silica is produced by drilling or processing rock such as granite or sandstone or when sand is used in sandblasting or foundry work.

Acute silicosis resulting from acute heavy exposure is rare but causes breathlessness and systemic upset over weeks with cyanosis and crackles on examination and widespread opacification on chest radiographs. Pulmonary testing is restrictive.

Silicotic nodularity on a chest radiograph, in contrast to pneumoconiosis, reflects intrapulmonary fibrotic nodules which develop as an exuberant response to scant dust that continues after exposure has ceased. Hilar glands may calcify and there is a predisposition to pulmonary tuberculosis.

Table 1 Occupational risk factors for the development of chronic airways obstruction

Coal mine dust	Asbestos
Cotton dust (byssinosis)	Grain and wood dusts
Welding fumes	Nitrogen oxides

Case history 17

A non-smoking farmer presented with a 14-month history of progressive breathlessness. His lung function was restrictive; his chest was unremarkable on examination with minimal changes on a chest radiograph. A high resolution CT scan was abnormal in keeping with extrinsic allergic alveolitis and bronchiolitis.

Thoughts?

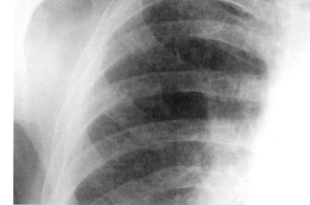

Fig. 3 **Chest radiograph demonstrating fine nodularity of simple pneumoconiosis.**

Occupational lung disease

- Always consider an occupational cause of lung disease and take a detailed occupational history in chronological order.

- Prevention of occupational lung disease is better than treatment. Prompt recognition and appropriate modification of work processes or practices are required to prevent further cases.

- Financial compensation may be due for some occupational disabilities.

INTERSTITIAL LUNG DISEASE

This is a heterogeneous group of diseases predominantly affecting the alveolar walls and septae, the parenchyma, in contrast to airways or vasculature. They are rare, though some may be becoming more common. In contrast to the few diseases of the airways, there are many interstitial lung diseases. They are usually first suspected when a chest radiograph demonstrates parenchymal shadowing.

All are characterised by inflammation, fibrosis or infiltration of lung parenchyma. The initial insult is usually at the alveolar wall, triggering inflammation and damage, an alveolitis, that may spill out into the airspaces and occasionally be associated with airway disease. The trigger may be recognised:

- asbestos and other fibrogenic dusts
- drugs, particularly amiodarone
- connective tissue diseases including rheumatoid.

In many other cases the stimulus is unknown. The lung infiltration, inflammation or resulting fibrosis is usually progressive and leads to lung rigidity and impaired compliance. Ventilatory capacity is usually restricted and may be obstructive.

This stiffness, coupled with stimulation of noiciceptive j-receptors within the lung parenchyma by the inflammatory process, leads to the early sensations of breathlessness and a non-productive cough. With progressive parenchymal loss, lung volumes fall and the stiff, small lungs become poor gas exchangers. Gas transfer is impaired as much by poor ventilation of abnormal but perfused lung as by alveolar–capillary thickening. Progressive hypoxia occurs, initially upon exercise or sleep. Ventilatory failure with hypercapnia and peripheral oedema occurs late. Disease progression is usually over a variable time scale of months to years. Occasionally, a more rampant decline occurs over weeks.

CLINICAL APPROACH

The clinical approach to the patient with progressive breathlessness and a dry cough where interstitial lung disease is a concern should include the following:

- A full drug history, including over-the-counter and herbal remedies.
- A detailed occupational and social history searching for exposures.
- Clinical evidence of other diseases, particularly connective tissue and malignancy.

- Physical examination that usually demonstrates restriction to chest expansion with lung crackles. Clubbing, and evidence of connective tissue diseases, should be sought.
- Laboratory investigations should include auto-antibodies, blood gas estimate and chest radiography.
- High resolution CT lung scanning is increasingly utilised. It provides further information on the parenchymal abnormalities and may suggest a location for either surgical or bronchoscopic lung biopsy. Increasingly, certain appearances with a high pathoradiological correlation obviate lung biopsy.
- Surgical lung biopsy is the diagnostic gold standard. Interpretation requires skilful integration of all the clinical and radiological information.

Therapy depends on a firm diagnosis ideally with biopsy support. It may involve respiratory protection or avoidance of exposures, drug cessation or a trial of steroids.

CRYPTOGENIC FIBROSING ALVEOLITIS (CFA)

This is an uncommon disease of the elderly with a male predominance. It may be becoming more prevalent. Though CFA clearly refers to pulmonary fibrosis without a recognisable cause, metal and wood dusts and previous viral infections may be considered triggers.

Clinical features

The characteristic feature is inspiratory crackles on auscultation at both lung bases. These may have been previously misinterpreted as heart failure or bronchitis. The patient develops finger clubbing with increasing restriction of chest expansion, and later develops central cyanosis and peripheral oedema. Pulmonary function testing confirms restriction with small lungs and impaired gas transfer. There may be circulating auto-antibodies and increased frequency of coincidental autoimmune disease.

The usual course is progressive exertional breathlessness with deteriorating lung function and exercise capacity. The median duration from diagnosis to death is 3.5 years. In some patients the decline is brisker over a few months with progressive fibrosis, termed Hamman–Rich syndrome.

Radiology

A chest radiograph shows reticular (lace-like) shadowing, predominantly at both lung bases. This is often symmetrical, and as it progresses the heart border appears increasingly indistinct ('ragged'). Lung fields are small and the honeycomb appearance of end-stage fibrosis becomes apparent.

High resolution CT lung scanning is useful. In early disease it is more sensitive than a plain chest radiograph. Later it can demonstrate patterns of fibrosis and characteristic opacification (Fig. 1).

Pathology

There are a range of abnormalities from recent neutrophil-rich inflammation extending into the alveoli through to collagen deposition and interstitial fibrosis. These appearances reflect a diffuse alveolar injury.

Therapy

Many patients are tried on high-dose corticosteroids. Immunosuppressive therapy is often added as 'steroid-sparing agents' to reduce the substantial effects of chronic oral steroid therapy in patients of this age-group. Though less than 40% of patients will respond with an objective improvement, even stemming a decline in lung function is a worthwhile achievement. Specific anti-fibrotic agents are now being explored and include colchicine and anti-cytokine preparations.

SARCOIDOSIS

Sarcoid is a multi-organ disease that may be asymptomatic or present non-specifically (Fig. 2). It is an immunological disorder associated with a characteristic histopathological feature of non-caseating granulomas. Though these are typical,

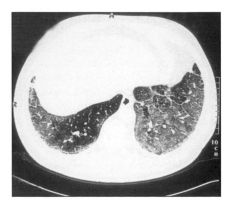

Fig. 1 **High resolution CT scan of the lung with ground glass and fibrosis.**

their presence requires the exclusion of tuberculosis and, if within the lungs, consideration of extrinsic allergic alveolitis or a drug reaction. Individuals of Caribbean black or Irish ethnic origins are more likely to develop the disease.

Sarcoid can affect any organ system but a pulmonary presentation is common.

- *Bilateral hilar lymphadenopathy (BHL)* (Fig. 3) may be asymptomatic but often accompanies an acute presentation with lethargy, joint aches and the skin rash of erythema nodosum, especially in young women. This acute presentation is the most benign form of sarcoid, when spontaneous resolution over a couple of years is typical. The most important differential diagnosis is lymphoma. A lateral chest radiograph is important as sarcoid adenopathy rarely fills the retrosternal space. BHL in patients from the Indian subcontinent may be tuberculosis.
- *Progressive pulmonary infiltrates,* typically midzone and subpleural, representing an alveolitis or fibrosis. They may occur in conjunction with, or independent of, BHL. There are extensive radiological changes but little on auscultation.
- *Bronchial mucosal infiltration* with a non-productive cough, rarely airways obstruction.
- *Cutaneous anergy to tuberculin PPD* as a Mantoux or Heaf test, even if prior BCG vaccination.

Diagnosis

When the clinical picture is characteristic, for instance BHL in a woman with erythema nodosum, the diagnosis is often self-evident. Serum immunoglobulins and angiotensin converting enzyme (ACE) levels can be measured as non-specific markers of disease activity. The serum ACE originates from active granulomata. In all other cases material is required for histological examination for the presence of non-caseating granulomas. Within the lungs, multiple bronchial biopsies are as likely to be positive as more peripheral lung biopsies. Occasionally, enlarged lymph nodes need to be excised to exclude the main clinical differential diagnosis of lymphoma. Mediastinal or hilar nodes will require mediastinoscopy. The Kveim test requires the intradermal injection of an extract of spleen from a patient with sarcoid and then biopsy of that skin site 6 weeks later examining for granulomata. It is losing popularity as other methods of confirmation are available and because of the risks of iatrogenic viral infection.

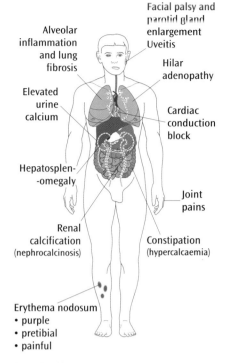

Fig. 2 **Manifestations of sarcoidosis.**

Facial palsy and parotid gland enlargement
Uveitis
Hilar adenopathy
Cardiac conduction block
Joint pains
Constipation (hypercalcaemia)
Renal calcification (nephrocalcinosis)
Hepatosplen-omegaly
Elevated urine calcium
Alveolar inflammation and lung fibrosis
Erythema nodosum
- purple
- pretibial
- painful

OTHER INTERSTITIAL LUNG DISEASES

Asbestosis is the result of inhaling substantial amounts of asbestos fibre over years. Even following cessation of exposure, fibrosis progresses though mortality is as likely to be due to an asbestos-related malignancy as to chronic respiratory failure. Chronic silica dust inhalation, as in hardrock mining, will cause pulmonary fibrosis.

An interstitial basal pulmonary fibrosis is associated with sero-positive rheumatoid arthritis and other connective tissue disorders.

Many drugs, including anti-inflammatory agents, can cause a range of interstitial lung diseases, including an acute toxic oedema, progressive interstitial pneumonitis or chronic inflammation with fibrosis. It is imperative to consider therapeutic and recreational drugs and other remedies as possible precipitants. The anti-arrhythmic amiodarone is the commonest drug causing pulmonary injury through both immunological and directly toxic mechanisms. Though to an extent

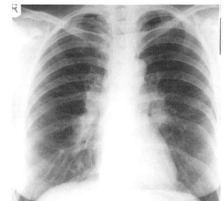

Fig. 3 **Plain chest X-ray with hilar node enlargement bilaterally.**

dependent on cumulative dose exposure, it can be difficult to recognise. There are characteristic cellular features and the iodine content of the retained drug causes radiodensity on CT lung imaging. Drug withdrawal may reverse some of the damage, but at risk of life-threatening cardiac dysrhythmias.

Chronic allergic alveolitis causes a more insidious breathlessness with radiological lung fibrosis and basal crackles on auscultation in contrast to acute allergen exposure. Beware the budgerigar in the living room corner and the tenant farmer with overwintering mouldy hay! Serological tests will confirm exposure but are not diagnostic of alveolitis. Avoidance of exposure with steroid therapy is the mainstay of treatment.

Case history 18

An overweight 50-year-old male presents with progressive breathlessness. Examination demonstrates lung crackles with bilateral infiltrates on a chest radiograph. High resolution CT scan demonstrates a predominantly midzone and nodular infiltrate. Thoracoscopic lung biopsy demonstrates a featureless quiescent fibrosis. Comment?

Interstitial lung disease

- Interstitial lung diseases are uncommon, predominantly parenchymal diseases characterised by progressive breathlessness, radiological infiltrates and, usually, restrictive physiology. There are many causes.
- A detailed history is required, including occupations, exposures and drug use.
- High resolution CT scan is most helpful, but lung biopsy is often required for a firm diagnosis.
- The mainstays of therapy are corticosteroids with immunosuppressant 'steroid-sparing' agents. More effective disease-modifying drugs are required.

OTHER INFLAMMATORY CONDITIONS

PULMONARY VASCULITIS

This is a rare heterogeneous group of disorders characterised by inflammation within the walls of blood vessels. The inflammatory process is likely to be driven by immune complexes that have leaked into the vessel wall due to abnormal endothelial permeability. There a cell-mediated immune response occurs with complement activation and local damage. Intravascular thrombosis due to endothelial damage contributes to the clinical consequences of vessel closure and tissue ischaemia or infarction. Some vasculitides are triggered by recognisable agents such as *Streptococcus* or hepatitis B virus, but for many forms of vasculitis no antigen has been implicated.

Pulmonary vasculitis is usually seen in the context of multisystem disorders. The clinical effects of pulmonary vasculitis may range from asymptomatic radiographic abnormalities to the lung taking the full brunt of the insult.

WEGENER'S GRANULOMATOSIS (WG)

This is the best example of a systemic vasculitis that has a range of consequences. It is becoming recognised more often and may becoming more common.

Pathology

The typical feature is inflammation extending through the full thickness of blood vessel walls, with the formation of necrotising granulomas. All blood vessels may be affected: a true angiitis.

Anti-neutrophil cytoplasmic antibodies (ANCAs)

These are IgG auto-antibodies directed against one of two constituents of neutrophil cytoplasm: either myeloperoxidase (termed p-ANCA from artefactual perinuclear staining on cell preparations) or protease-3 (cytoplasmic staining, c-ANCA). ANCAs have been recognised as a characteristic serum auto-antibody detectable in nearly 90% of patients with active WG, especially c-ANCA which in high titre is closely associated with WG. Low levels of c-ANCA or the presence of p-ANCA is less specific, being present in other vasculitides and even non-vasculitic diseases.

These auto-antibodies are likely to be involved in the pathogenesis of WG. They are able to activate neutrophils and are directly toxic to vascular endothelium. The disease appears to be driven from within the lungs where there are higher levels of these antibodies in broncho-alveolar fluid than in peripheral blood. With effective treatment, c-ANCA levels usually fall and may rise months before a clinically apparent relapse.

Clinical features

This rare condition affects middle-aged people with an equal sex incidence. It is becoming more common, not solely due to the ability to detect ANCAs. Increasing exposure of the population to an inhaled trigger(s) such as oil seed rape has been suggested.

The most frequently involved system is the respiratory tract (Fig. 1). The lungs are involved in more then 80% of cases and at presentation in nearly half.

The next most commonly involved organ is the kidney with a proliferative glomerulonephritis on renal biopsy and associated with a poorer outlook. Microscopic haematuria with cellular casts on urine microscopy will progress if untreated to renal failure requiring dialysis.

Other organs involved less commonly include the skin (with a vasculitic rash) (Fig. 2), eyes with retro-orbital masses, gut with infarcts and perforation and cerebritis. Non-specific peripheral blood abnormalities of acute inflammation are present with a leucocytosis, a mild normochromic anaemia and elevated acute phase reactants. There is usually evidence of multi-system involvement even at presentation. However, WG may rarely remain a single organ disease affecting solely the lungs or kidney.

Treatment

Untreated the disease is fatal. Corticosteroids alone are inadequate. Immunosuppression with both steroids and cyclophosphamide is usual with careful titration of therapy over many months to clinical evidence of disease activity supported by ANCA titres. Using such a regime, disease remission is achieved in a median of 12 months. However, this treatment is associated with appreciable toxicity. This includes both haemorrhagic cystitis and infertility due to the cyclophosphamide; infections due to both agents with osteoporosis and malignancy are longer term effects.

Alternative treatment regimes are being developed. Azathioprine is often substituted for the cyclophosphamide after an induction period of several months. Etoposide and methotrexate have been used; and co-trimoxazole may be useful in sinusitis. Plasma exchange has a role in rapidly progressive renal failure or lung haemorrhage.

OTHER VASCULITIDES

Allergic granulomatosis with angiitis or Churg–Strauss syndrome

This involves asthma often with rhinitis developing in middle-aged patients. Over months to years a peripheral blood

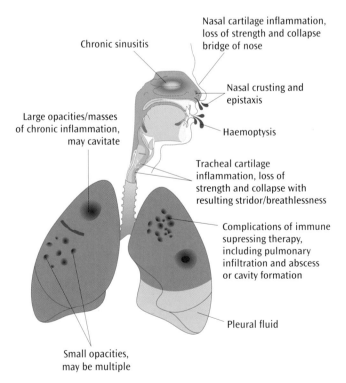

Fig. 1 **Respiratory consequences of Wegener's granulomatosis.**

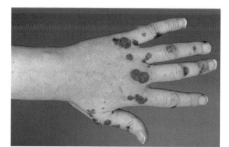

Fig. 2 **Skin vasculitis.**

eosinophilia becomes prominent together with a fever and variable infiltrates on chest radiographs. The final clinical phase of the disease is a life-threatening systemic vasculitis. Cardiac involvement is frequent and a cause of death; by contrast clinical evidence of renal involvement is rare. The systemic vasculitis is usually very steroid responsive.

Small vessel vasculitides

Small vessel angiitis can result in radiographic infiltrates, haemoptysis or alveolar haemorrhage. It is often associated with systemic diseases such as Henoch–Schönlein purpura or polyarteritis nodosa. Treatment of the underlying disease or with steroids usually produces a good response.

Polyangiitis overlap syndrome

This is a term reserved for a systemic vasculitis that cannot be otherwise categorised. Pulmonary involvement may occur if the overlap includes features of either granulomatous pulmonary vasculitis or asthma with pulmonary eosinophil infiltration. Immunosuppression with steroids and another agent, as for Wegener's granulomatosis, is usually required.

Pulmonary vasculitis and connective tissue disorders

Rheumatoid arthritis

Though there are many common pleuro-pulmonary manifestations of rheumatoid arthritis, pulmonary vasculitis is rare. It occurs in patients who are sero-positive with extra-articular disease. It is suspected when a patient develops pulmonary hypertension out of proportion to known parenchymal lung disease and peripheral oxygenation. Specific treatment is difficult. There is little evidence of benefit with steroids or immunosuppressive therapy. Anticoagulants and domiciliary oxygen therapy are often tried as palliative measures.

Systemic sclerosis

Pulmonary vasculitis with unexplained pulmonary hypertension can be an early feature of the variant CREST that comprises subcutaneous calcific deposits, peripheral digital vasospasm, swallowing difficulties and facial skin changes. There maybe therapeutic benefit from selected vasodilators (nifedipine).

Other connective tissue diseases

Systemic lupus erythematosus (SLE) is very rarely associated with pulmonary vasculitis. A small vessel angiitis may result in alveolar haemorrhage that responds to steroids. Behçet's disease may be associated with vasculitic pulmonary vessel closure and subsequent lung infarction with pleurisy, haemoptysis and radiographic pleural-based infiltrates.

ALVEOLAR HAEMORRHAGE

Intrapulmonary haemorrhage can be life threatening or clinically silent except for a progressive iron-deficiency anaemia. Usually haemoptysis is associated with breathlessness and non-specific alveolar shadowing on a chest radiograph that may be mistaken for pulmonary oedema. Haemoptysis may range from streaking to substantial amounts and the respiratory embarrassment may result in ventilatory failure. Occasionally there is no haemoptysis and rarely no radiographic abnormality at times of alveolar bleeding.

Lung function testing may show a restrictive defect. The characteristic abnormality is an elevated transfer factor for carbon monoxide gas which is taken up avidly by the intrapulmonary haemoglobin. In ill patients a single breath gas transfer measurement is difficult to obtain.

Lung biopsy or alveolar fluid sampling by broncho-alveolar lavage 48 hours or more following haemorrhage will demonstrate degraded haemoglobin (haemosiderin) within alveolar macrophages from ingested erythrocytes.

There are a number of causes:

When associated with renal failure

In Goodpasture's syndrome, there is often a recognised trigger such as a viral illness or contact with volatile chemicals. A circulating antibody directed against a glomerular basement membrane collagen (anti-GBM) is generated. This is deposited in glomerulae and in alveolar capillaries too. Here it initiates immunologically mediated damage that results in a rampant glomerulonephritis, renal failure and lung haemorrhage without pulmonary vasculitis. Organ support, immunosuppression and plasma exchange are required.

Other pulmonary vasculitides or connective tissue diseases may be associated with progressive renal failure and alveolar haemorrhage. Clearly, anti-GBM antibodies are absent but other auto-antibodies such as anti-nuclear or ANCAs may be present.

Without associated renal failure

There is a range of causes including chronically elevated pulmonary venous pressure by mitral valve stenosis, pulmonary emboli with infarction, coagulopathy from primary haematological disorders or anticoagulant therapy and rarely drug therapy.

Case history 19

A male patient with poorly controlled hypertension presents with a short history of fever and haemoptysis. He is taking oral anticoagulants for atrial fibrillation and is known to have chronic renal impairment. When examined he is in modest respiratory distress, crackles were audible over both lung fields and bilateral infiltrates present on a chest radiograph. Early investigations suggest acute deterioration of chronic renal impairment.

What diagnostic possibilities spring to mind and how might you proceed?

Other inflammatory conditions

- Pulmonary vasculitis is rare, usually occurring in the context of a multi-system upset.
- Wegener's granulomatosis is a potentially life-threatening vasculitis and patients may present to a number of specialists. Inflammation without infection particularly in the face of renal abnormalities should raise suspicions.
- The ability to test for anti-neutrophil antibodies (ANCAs) has undoubtedly helped in the diagnosis of WG, but beware of over-interpreting low titres especially p-ANCA in unusual clinical settings.

ASTHMA I

Asthma is the clinical result of a chronic eosinophil-rich inflammation of the bronchial tree. Although the mechanisms of both disease onset and subsequent exacerbations are incompletely understood, there has been much recent progress in our understanding.

EPIDEMIOLOGY AND PATHOGENESIS

Asthma is one of the commonest chronic diseases in the developed world. It affects 10–15% of children and 5–10% of adults at least. Epidemiological studies from differing continents suggest that it is becoming truly more prevalent, as well as being better recognised. The development of asthma in any one individual seems to be due to interaction between the environment and a genetic predisposition. Epidemiological studies implicate as environmental influences:

- early exposure to airborne allergens such as house dust mite faeces, tobacco smoke, air pollutants
- peri- or pre-natal factors incompletely identified but include maternal smoking, diet including sodium content and antioxidants.

The genetic component is unlikely to be a single gene abnormality but rather polygenic. Gene candidates for disturbed function may include:

- IgE receptors and subunits
- β_2 adrenoreceptor genes.

Asthma is an important cause of morbidity and mortality with appreciable social and financial costs to individuals, families and society (Table 1). There is an appreciable mortality due to asthma with over 2000 patients, many young, dying each year in the UK. Epidemics of asthma deaths occurred in many developed countries in the 1960s and again in the late 1980s. The earlier epidemic was probably related to an over-reliance on the newly available inhaled non-selective β-agonist therapy and under-utilised prophylaxis (Fig. 1). The later deaths were in part due to the type of β_2-agonist therapy used, especially in Australasia. Fortunately, these rates are now beginning to fall in many countries.

IMMUNOPATHOLOGY

Mucosal biopsies and pathological specimens from patients with asthma demonstrate inflammatory changes throughout the bronchial wall. The epithelium is damaged or shed, the basement membrane may be thickened and in chronic asthma fibrosis may have occurred. The submucosa is oedematous with vascular engorgement and leakage. Within the mucosa there an inflammatory cell infiltrate rich in eosinophils and lymphocytes generating a soup of pro-inflammatory cytokines. Many of these lymphocytes are of the T_{h2} subset attracting eosinophils. These eosinophils release pro-inflammatory and cytotoxic products that maintain a vicious cycle of inflammation and cell damage. There is also neuro-humeral interaction with neurogenic inflammation, release of nitric oxide and cytokine irritation of sensitised nerve endings. The airway smooth muscle is hypertrophied and in spasm with defective β_2-receptor driven muscle relaxation.

Even in clinically quiescent asthma, persisting inflammation may lead to altered airway structure with subepithelial fibrosis resulting in irreversible limitation to airflow. This remodelling is less readily reversed with therapy and may be less amenable to the development of novel target-directed therapies than acute inflammatory pathways.

PATHOPHYSIOLOGY

A range of inhaled irritants leads to airway epithelial shedding, inflammatory mucosal oedema, smooth muscle contraction and increased secretions. As a result of this bronchial wall inflammation, airways narrow easily in response to a wide range of stimuli, including many non-specific insults such as cold air. This is an exaggeration of normal and is termed bronchial 'hyper-responsiveness' or 'hyper-reactivity'. Continuing inflammation directly and indirectly via bronchial hyper-reactivity causes persisting though variable symptoms of asthma. If this occurs on a background of chronic bronchial wall inflammation and muscle contraction, very little further reduction in airway calibre is needed to produce a marked clinically apparent increase in resistance to airflow (flow $\propto$ calibre^4) (Fig. 2).

Expiratory flow in particular is impaired as airways are normally further narrowed in expiration. In patients experiencing deteriorating asthma, a wheeze reflecting turbulent airflow through these narrowed airways may be audible, initially on expiration and with worsening resistance on inspiration too. This is reflected in a marked reduction in FEV_1 and PEFR as bedside measures of airway geometry. Forced vital capacity is also reduced in part due to early closure on expiration of narrowed airways with air trapping developing as dynamic hyperventilation.

In the early stages of an exacerbation there is reflex overventilation with lowering of arterial pCO_2. As the resistance to airflow increases, with mucous plugs and oedematous bronchial walls, the pressures required and the associated work of breathing increase substantially. This required increase in respiratory work and associated minute volume is in the face of an increasing mechanical disadvantage imposed on the respiratory muscles by the hyperinflation. Adverse metabolic changes including hypo-kalaemia and anaerobic metabolism may further impair respiratory muscle performance.

Accordingly, arterial pO_2 falls due to the perfusion of relatively hypoxic underventilated lung units, hypoxaemia that is usually readily responsive to oxygen therapy. Arterial pCO_2 begins to rise due to a combination of respiratory muscle fatigue with failing ventilation and an inability to generate the required increase in minute ventilation to clear the carbon dioxide generated by the respiratory muscles. Mechanical ventilatory support may then be required to control the CO_2 and associated acidosis. With further airway narrowing, and plugging, respiratory failure, hypoxic confusion, coma and cardiac arrest may ensue. Spontaneous recovery or response to therapy arrests and reverses this potential spiral of deterioration.

CLINICAL FEATURES

Asthma can arise at any age, though onset in childhood is more likely to be recognised as asthma than onset in the elderly. Childhood asthma is usually atopic, an 'allergic tendency' to 'extrin-

Table 1 **The costs of asthma**

Health service	£4.9 x10^8 NHS drug bill (1995–6) consultant/GP/nurse time 110 432 admissions (1993)
Society	17 x 10^6 days lost (1994–5)* £3.4 x 10^8 lost production (1990)*
	Sleep disturbance (school or work underperformance) Childhood asthma (learning and family disruption) Death 1665 (1994) (what price?)

* likely to be under-certificated

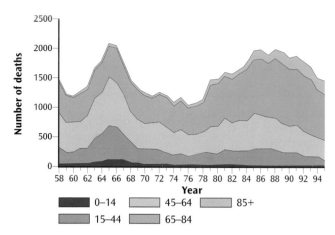

Fig. 1 **Deaths coded as asthma, England and Wales 1958–1995.** Note how two peaks have occurred—the first among young people and the second among the elderly. Changes in coding have occurred during this period. (Source: Office of National Statistics.)

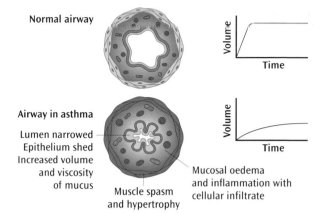

Fig. 2 **Normal and asthmatic airways in cross-section.**

sic' precipitants and associated with eczema, seasonal rhinitis or migraine. Later onset of asthma may be a resurgence of childhood atopy. Alternatively, onset may be triggered by viral infections or other factors without atopic associations ('intrinsic').

Symptoms are usually intermittent at the outset, though may become persistent with delayed or under-treatment. They typically consist of:

- cough; usually dry, sometimes productive of even purulent sputum (usually reflecting inflammation rather than infection)
- breathlessness
- wheeze
- chest tightness, discomfort and even pain.

Many of these symptoms are worse at night, reflecting increased diurnal variation of airway calibre and probably inflammation. Signs such as wheeze on chest auscultation and objective measures of airflow limitation such as PEFR will vary too. Between exacerbations, such clinical assessment may be quite normal but does not disprove asthma as the diagnosis, nor does it confirm that the underlying inflammatory mechanisms are suppressed.

This variability of symptoms and signs may occur over a short time scale, typically overnight or following exercise. Exacerbations over longer periods may be precipitated by upper respiratory tract viral infections or more chronic exposures including occupational precipitants. Common exacerbating factors include:

- diurnal, early morning or nocturnal worsening with sleep disturbance and poor daytime performance
- exercise

- environmental:
  - tobacco smoke
  - temperature or weather changes, thunderstorms
  - paint, perfume, fumes
  - air pollutants: ozone, particulates, oxides of sulphur and nitrogen
- infections: viral (hardly ever bacterial)
- drugs: aspirin, other NSAIDs, β blockers (even topical)
- immunological:
  - house dust mite aero-allergens
  - pollens, seasonal
  - platinum salts, Western red cedar wood dust
- psyche: emotional upset,

Such variability of symptoms and signs is crucial in establishing a diagnosis of asthma. All that wheezes is not asthma though. Look for generalised wheeze (not endobronchial obstruction from tumour or foreign body), airflow limitation with variability or reversibility on therapy. Other causes of airways obstruction include COPD, bronchiectasis and obliterative bronchiolitis.

The exaggerated bronchial response to these precipitants with associated symptoms and signs reflect bronchial hyper-responsiveness. However, direct measurement of hyper-responsiveness to inhalational challenge is rarely required in routine clinical practice. It can be measured by the response in airway calibre (change FEV_1 or airway resistance) to inhaled non-specific broncho-constrictors methacholine or histamine. It is a useful measurement only when clinical doubt remains over a diagnosis of asthma, in the assessment of occupational asthma, in epidemiological studies and in drug evaluation or research.

Case history 20

A school boy is brought by his parents because of a regular night-time cough that is keeping the rest of the family awake. He is unaware of this but feels tired during the day and avoids sports and gym because he is 'unfit'.

Could this be asthma ?

How would you confirm it ?

Asthma I

- Asthma is the commonest chronic disease in the western world and is probably becoming commoner.
- The important clinical features are of generalised airways obstruction that is variable in time or reversible with adequate therapy.
- Even careful clinical assessment may under-recognise the degree of bronchial inflammation. Persisting unrelieved inflammation leads to structural airway changes.

ASTHMA II

PSYCHOLOGICAL ASPECTS

The psychopathological and psychosocial aspects of individuals with asthma is increasingly appreciated. Patients with any severe or recurrent disease may develop denial behaviours as a coping strategy to limit the intrusion of the disease and its management into their lifestyle. Other patients with severe asthma may have a blunted perception of breathlessness. If asthma then worsens, these factors may delay their ability to respond before the attack becomes life threatening. Such issues should be explored in patients with recurrent or near-fatal attacks of asthma. It also underlines the need for management to be based on objective measures of severity.

Psychosocial issues are relevant in the management of any patient with asthma. Interaction with family members, work or school associates and healthcare workers are all opportunities for intervention, friction or manipulation. Many patients on daily therapy will question the need for regular therapy and choose to balance such commitment against respiratory symptoms that may include sleep disturbance. Although their disease may appear not completely controlled, patients feel an increased sense of control, though at the risk of being viewed as non-compliers.

NON-PHARMACOLOGICAL THERAPY

Avoidance of exacerbating factors is not always possible. Avoiding animal hair may lead to interpersonal stresses if the offending animal is not the patient's own. House dust mite is impossible to eradicate from centrally heated housing and measures to reduce airborne allergen load sufficient to improve pulmonary function are draconian. Patients living in damp housing may be able to be rehoused.

Stopping smoking and avoiding passive smoke is a vital and achievable aspect of therapy. Professional carers should be the advocate of young patients if parents persist in smoking.

Air pollution is topical though the evidence that it *causes* asthma is lacking. Exacerbations may be precipitated by high levels of air pollution which may be predictable. Patients whose asthma is known to deteriorate during such episodes should temporarily increase their prophylactic therapy. Certain herbal remedies help some patients some of the time. The evidence for a consistent benefit

attributable to air ionisers or acupuncture is lacking, though on an individual basis may be worth pursuing.

Communication with and education of the patient and carers is crucial. They should have a basic understanding of asthma and its treatment, be able to recognise the symptoms of deteriorating control, know what action to take and have such an action plan in writing. They may also have a peak flow meter and modify their therapy accordingly. Such co-management improves morbidity, reducing emergency contacts.

PHARMACOLOGICAL THERAPY

Principles of therapy

The goals of therapy are to abolish day- and night-time symptoms, to achieve and maintain best possible lung function and minimise deterioration with associated disruption of family, school and work. Anti-inflammatory therapy is the mainstay of therapy, used promptly and aggressively to gain symptom control and reversal of airways obstruction before easing to maintenance therapy. It is becoming apparent that measures of bronchial inflammation, such as inflammatory markers in induced sputum rather than of airway geometry should be the monitor of therapy.

Drug delivery

Most asthma therapy is inhaled in small doses directly to the lungs to maximise the therapeutic effect and minimise unwanted side-effects. Subsequent absorption into the pulmonary vascular bed may still be an important factor in causing systemic effects. The selection of a device for drug delivery involves patient participation, especially if young or with arthritis.

The means of drug delivery include:

- **Metered-dose pressurised aerosol inhaler (MDI).** These use CFC or non-CFC propellants to deliver a particulate dose ejected at high velocity. The device has changed little in 40 years and is difficult to use competently by both adults and children. The most challenging aspect in its use is the co-ordination of activation with deep inspiration. This problem of co-ordination can be remedied by using either an MDI with a large volume spacer or an Autohaler that senses inspiration and automatically delivers the dose. Devices that improve pulmonary

deposition by slowing the aerosol velocity in a vortex still require co-ordination with patient inspiration.

- **Dry powder delivery devices (DPI).** These require inhalation through a device to entrain and deliver microcrystalline drug into the lungs. They are easier to use than an MDI but tend to be more expensive and are not available for all drugs.

- **Nebulisers.** These deliver mists of aqueous drug particles generated by passing either high flow oxygen or air through the drug solution. A range of particle sizes are produced. An appropriate nebulisation chamber will filter particle size and increase the proportion of respirable particles delivered. The equipment is not cheap but is portable and may be the only device for small children. Drugs that can be nebulised include bronchodilators, steroids and certain antibiotics.

- **Oral administration of drugs.** This is simple, often cheap and is favoured by many patients.

- **Parenteral delivery.** This is useful as a short-term measure of delivering β_2-agonists when patients are mechanically ventilated with airways resistance unresponsive to conventional aggressive therapy. Aminophylline is administered by infusions. The extremely rare patient with very labile asthma may respond to continuous subcutaneous infusions of β-agonists.

Drug therapy

Anti-inflammatory agents

Steroids

Topically potent glucocorticoids are the mainstay of treatment: there are as yet no targeted anti-inflammatory drugs of comparable efficacy. Inhaled steroids reduce bronchial inflammation and produce a measurable improvement in symptoms and airway function over 10–14 days.

Effective therapy prevents exacerbations, sleep disruption and reduces hospital attendances. Bronchial hyper-reactivity is normalised over several months. Some of the adverse structural airway changes of under-controlled asthma may also be reversed. Deposition of inhaled steroid on the oropharynx may cause oral candidiasis and voice changes. Systemic side-effects may occur when high doses or highly potent drugs are inhaled and either absorbed across the pulmonary bed or when the oropharyngeal deposit is swallowed, absorbed and is incompletely extracted by the liver. Oral steroid therapy is required in severe exacerbations (Fig. 1) and may be required at other times to gain rapid control of symptoms. If asthma remains chronically severe, then the addition of lowest dose oral steroid therapy may be required. The aim should be to minimise if not stop the oral therapy at the earliest opportunity.

Non-steroidal anti-inflammatory drugs
Sodium chromoglycate and nedocromil have a role as an alternative to steroids, the former having a place in the treatment of children. Anti-inflammatory agents that are more selective than steroids are becoming available, such as leukotriene (LT) β-antagonists. The redundancy of pro-inflammatory pathways would suggest only a modest benefit will be obtained and the early clinical experience supports that. There is increasing evidence that chronic therapy with oral methylxanthines at doses lower than that considered conventional for bronchodilation may have an anti-inflammatory effect. There is a little experience of methotrexate and cyclosporin as steroid-sparing agents in chronic severe asthma where these drugs are used to minimise the daily steroid dose but are not without appreciable side-effects.

Bronchodilators
β$_2$-agonists when inhaled directly cause airway smooth muscle relaxation within minutes and lasting for 4–5 hrs. Side-effects include tremor and tachycardia. When nebulised at high dose and with oral steroids there is the risk of hypokalaemia and cardiac dysrrhythmia.

Long acting β$_2$-agonist inhaled agents provide 12–18 hours' cover which is especially useful overnight and to prevent exercise-induced symptoms during the day. They may have an additional steroid-sparing effect though the mechanism is unclear.

Anticholinergic agents block pre-synaptic muscarinic receptors, thus relaxing airway smooth muscles. Their effect is in addition to the relaxation provided by β-agonists alone.

Methylxanthines, including caffeine, theophyllines and aminophylline, have been recognised as bronchodilators probably via adenosine antagonism.

Novel drugs
More specific anti-T-cell drugs and monoclonal antibodies that block IgE action have been developed and are

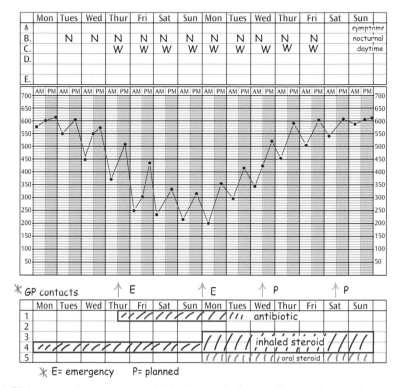

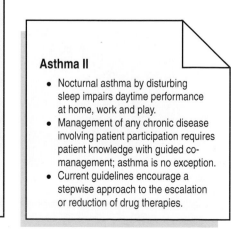

Fig 1 **Clinical course through an exacerbation, demonstrating effective use of aggressive anti-inflammatory therapy and demands in terms of night and day symptoms and medical contacts.**

currently being tested. Magnesium sulphate has bronchodilatory activity, probably by blocking intracellular calcium channels allowing airway smooth muscle relaxation. There are anecdotal reports of benefit though formal trials in mild to moderately severe acute asthma have failed to demonstrate a benefit additional to standard therapies. It is probably worth trying as a last resort prior to mechanical ventilation in very severe asthma.

Practical aspects
Diagnosis of asthma rests on the demonstration of variability in airflow obstruction. The objective response to inhaled or nebulised bronchodilators over minutes, or the effect of inhaled or oral steroids over weeks can be essential. A lack of response at a time when tests of airflow limitation are normal is unhelpful.

Therapeutic consensus has now developed with national guidelines and local protocols. They offer advice for the management of all phases of asthma and undergo periodic revision. Severe episodes require therapy with nebulised bronchodilators, steroids and oxygen with repeated objective reassessments. Chronic therapy can be approached in a stepwise fashion, moving up or down the therapeutic ladder with the patient in control.

Case history 21

A teenager with asthma was referred to a hospital clinic as he has poor asthma control despite an increasing dose of inhaled steroid and additional medications. He is seen first by a respiratory nurse specialist. The patient's preferred delivery device is identified, its use demonstrated and a correct delivery technique developed. 1 month later he is seen again with improved asthma control and he is taking a lower total daily dose of inhaled steroid.

Asthma II

- Nocturnal asthma by disturbing sleep impairs daytime performance at home, work and play.
- Management of any chronic disease involving patient participation requires patient knowledge with guided co-management; asthma is no exception.
- Current guidelines encourage a stepwise approach to the escalation or reduction of drug therapies.

CHRONIC OBSTRUCTIVE PULMONARY DISEASE (COPD) I

Previously variable and confusing terms for tobacco-induced chronic lung disease had included chronic obstructive airways or pulmonary disease (COAD, COLD), chronic airflow limitation or chronic airways obstruction. The term chronic obstructive pulmonary disease (COPD) is now standard in North America and the UK. It is a major source of disability and ill-health with many primary care attendances and hospital admissions due to this disease spectrum (Table 1).

CHRONIC BRONCHITIS

Chronic bronchitis is defined clinically as the presence of a productive cough most days of the month, for three consecutive months on two consecutive years. The majority of tobacco smokers meet this criterion as a result of the non-specific irritant effects of inhaled smoke. This irritation causes hyperplasia of bronchial epithelial goblet cells and mucosal glands which in turn secrete increased amounts of mucus. Tobacco smoke also reduces the effectiveness of the mucociliary escalator and, in conjunction with intercurrent infection, increased amounts of viscid secretions are produced and require to be expectorated.

Other inhaled irritants can result in a chronic productive cough. In Bombay, chronic bronchitis in cigarette smokers is prevalent a decade younger than in west European smokers, probably because of differences in particulate air pollution. Upon cessation of exposure to the irritant, sputum production may dwindle.

EMPHYSEMA

By contrast, emphysema is defined pathologically as the destruction of alveolar walls with consequent dilation of alveoli sacs. The advent of computed tomography, particularly high resolution CT scans (Fig.

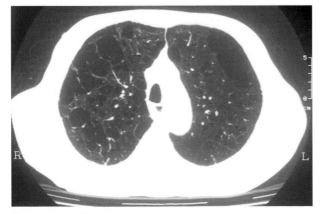

Fig. 1 **High resolution CT scan.**

Table 1 **Risk factors other than tobacco smoking for the development of chronic airways obstruction**

Occupational	Non-occupational
• Coal mine dust	• Early childhood LRTIs
• Asbestos	• Socio-economic
• Cotton dust (byssinosis)	• Diet
• Grain and wood dusts	• Anti-oxidants
• Welding fumes	• Air pollution
• Nitrogen oxides	

1), has allowed the easier recognition of emphysema in life. On such scans, air-containing apparently wall-less cysts are visible representing macroscopic dilated emphysematous airspaces.

The mechanism of parenchymal destruction has not been entirely established. Inhaled tobacco smoke causes chronic inflammation driven by alveolar macrophages, especially at the level of the terminal bronchioles. As part of this inflammation, neutrophils are attracted into the airways and lung interstitium and sequester in the pulmonary microvasculature. These cells are activated and release a range of tissue-damaging chemicals. The released proteolytic enzymes (especially elastase) are usually counterbalanced by serum and tissue anti-proteases. This protective screen is susceptible to inactivation either by reactive oxidising chemicals released from activated leucocytes or by active oxidant molecules contained in freshly inhaled cigarette smoke. The long-term balance between, on the one hand, unrestrained proteolytic activity which results in lung elastin destruction and, on the other, anti-protease defences is important in determining the development of emphysema.

In the 20–30% of heavy smokers who develop emphysema, a repetitive yet net imbalance favouring lung elastin destruction occurs over many years. It is not clear why only a minority of smokers develop emphysema. A very few of these susceptible smokers are deficient in the major protective protease inhibitor, alpha-1 antitrypsin or alpha-1 protease inhibitor (α_1Pi). The mechanisms of susceptibility in the remaining cigarette smokers who develop emphysema in the presence of normal α_1Pi levels are unclear but may relate to functional deficiencies in other anti-proteases or in anti-oxidant protection.

Alpha-1 protease inhibitor (α_1Pi) deficiency

In the early 1960s, a few patients who had demonstrated increased susceptibility to cigarette smoke by developing premature pulmonary emphysema were discovered to have deficient serum levels of α_1 anti-trypsin. Since then more than 70 variations in molecular form of the anti-protease now termed α_1Pi have been discovered and are inherited as autosomal co-dominant. Very few are associated with susceptibility to cigarette smoke and premature emphysema. In western Europe the majority of people display the normal MM type.

Barely 0.03% of the population are genotype ZZ. These individuals have a single amino acid change in the α_1Pi molecule. This alters the protein's final structure so the liver is unable to secrete the synthesised α_1Pi which accumulates intracellularly. The serum activity is barely a third of normal and some patients present with liver disease in childhood. Others miss developing chronic liver disease but, if cigarette smokers, present with premature mixed panacinar and centrilobular emphysema. In non-smokers the deficiency is compatible with normal life expectation and lung function, though there is an increased risk of chronic bronchial sepsis. Gene therapy can now temporarily raise levels of α_1Pi in the lungs though there have been no long-term trials demonstrating effective protection or preservation of lung function. Patients with heterozygous (MZ) or other α_1Pi phenotypes may have low–normal serum activities but are not unduly susceptible to developing emphysema.

COPD: STRICTLY DEFINED

The term 'chronic bronchitis and emphysema' is often used synonymously for COPD. However, the term COPD is limited to those individuals, often smokers who develop chronic and poorly reversible airways obstruction. The patient may be symptom-free in the early stages but as airways obstruction progresses, respiratory reserve is steadily eroded until breathlessness, initially on exertion, is noticed. This progresses relentlessly with increasing disability (Table 1).

The term should not be used for the fully reversible airways obstruction of asthma. However, the term may be loosely applied to patients with long-standing irreversible asthma, especially if they smoke. It clearly excludes the small number of

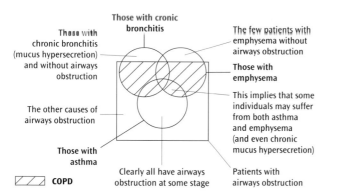

Fig. 2 **Overlapping relationship between chronic bronchitis (clinical), emphysema (clinico-radiological and pathology) and asthma (clinical) with COPD.** (After the original Venn diagram by G. Snider.)

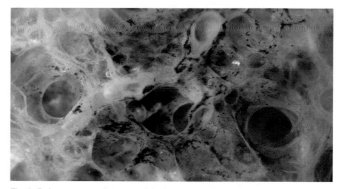

Fig. 3 **Pulmonary emphysema with airway loss of supports.**

breathless smokers with emphysema who do not have airways obstruction (Fig. 2).

Airways limitation

Airway obstruction in asthma is readily understandable on the basis of inflammatory mucosal oedema, mucus secretion and muscle spasm. No one of these factors is singularly important in the airflow limitation of COPD. Rather, it is the destruction of the elastin-containing alveolar walls supporting the small airways as emphysema develops (Fig. 3), compounded by bronchiolar inflammation and fibrosis consequent on chronic cigarette smoking. Poorly supported, these small airways narrow and tend to collapse, especially on expiration. Attempts at forced expiration will worsen this tendency. Airway narrowing and premature closure combined with the lack of elastic recoil consequent on elastin loss lead to distal air trapping and consequent lung overexpansion (Fig. 4).

Natural history

There is a natural decline in FEV_1 and peak flow with age, substantiated mainly by studies cross-sectional in time rather than large longitudinal studies. Non-smokers and smokers not susceptible to the airways obstructing effects of tobacco lose about 30 ml per year from their FEV_1. Susceptible smokers lose volume nearly twice as quickly. If smokers start at a young age they might never achieve their full pulmonary potential in their twenties and, if susceptible, lose lung function from a lower starting point (Fig. 5). Individual smokers may lose function in a stuttering manner with periods of stability even at poor levels of pulmonary function.

Unfortunately, there is no test to predict susceptibility to tobacco smoke except the accelerated loss of lung function. Recent data suggests that following smoking cessation, lung function may actually improve for a few years before declining to parallel that of the non-smoker. Attempts to quit early are crucial to delay the onset of disability: maximising disability-free years.

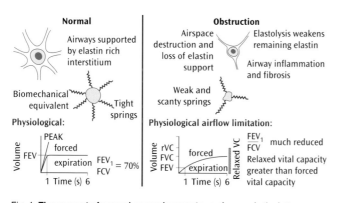

Fig. 4 **The support of normal or emphysematous airways.** In the latter, insufficient and poorly elastic supports result in premature collapse and airways obstruction, hence airflow limitation.

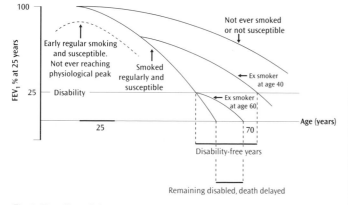
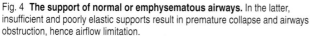

Fig. 5 **The effect of cigarette smoking, susceptibility and lung function decline.** (After Fletcher & Peto 1977; reproduced with permission from the BMJ.)

Case history 22

A 66-year-old male, a smoker of 20–30/day since teens with a daily productive cough for at least 10 years now presents with a few years of progressive exertional breathlessness without variability. With a spirometer you record an FEV_1 54% predicted and a FEV/VC ratio 50%. What is the likely diagnosis and why?

He re-presents 18 months later with heaviness deep in his left chest and a change in his cough, now irritating day and night. He is still smoking. What do you do now?

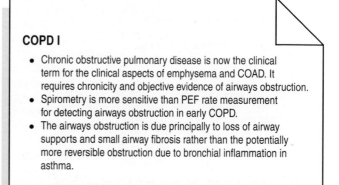

COPD I

- Chronic obstructive pulmonary disease is now the clinical term for the clinical aspects of emphysema and COAD. It requires chronicity and objective evidence of airways obstruction.
- Spirometry is more sensitive than PEF rate measurement for detecting airways obstruction in early COPD.
- The airways obstruction is due principally to loss of airway supports and small airway fibrosis rather than the potentially more reversible obstruction due to bronchial inflammation in asthma.

CHRONIC OBSTRUCTIVE PULMONARY DISEASE (COPD) II

CLINICAL FEATURES

The cardinal clinical features are:
- progressive breathlessness, sometimes with variability
- current or past tobacco smoking
- objective evidence of airways obstruction.

A discrete event such as a respiratory infection may precipitate a medical contact. They will have a long current or previous history of tobacco smoking often with symptoms of chronic bronchitis.

There may be little abnormal to find on examination. Conversely, the patient may be noticeably breathless with prolonged expiration through pursed lips and a hyper-expanded chest. The anterior–posterior thoracic expansion is diminished on respiration. The apparent paradox of voluntarily increasing resistance to expiration through pursed lips is an attempt to increase intra-airway pressure, reducing airway closure and airways obstruction. A cardinal sign of airflow limitation is the presence of intercostal indrawing during inspiration. A wheeze may be audible. In addition, on physical examination, complications of other tobacco-related diseases may be apparent.

CONFIRMING AIRWAYS OBSTRUCTION

Spirometry or a peak-flow meter are readily available techniques for measuring airways obstruction. A dry seal spirometer that measures expired volume directly is the ideal technique to measure FEV_1 and FVC. In airway obstruction, FEV_1 is more affected than FVC, though as the obstruction worsens forced VC falls. This is in part due to air trapping behind the airways closing on forced expiration and in part to such prolongation of expiration beyond the 6 seconds of the test. In such patients a slow relaxed expiratory effort will yield a greater expired VC. Modern portable hand-held spirometers measure flow directly, which is then integrated against time for volume. Unfortunately, many patients with severe COPD produce such low expiratory flow rates as to cause significant error with these devices.

Peak flow meters are readily available. However, in COPD the peak expiratory flow is relatively well preserved compared to FEV_1. Hence, it is not so useful for the early detection of airways obstruction when interventions to prevent disease progression might expect to be more successful.

VARIABILITY OF AIRWAYS OBSTRUCTION

The airways obstruction of COPD is typically poorly reversible as a result of the structural lung damage. However, in managing patients, absolute nihilism cannot reign: attempts must be made to minimise elements of obstruction due to airway smooth muscle constriction, mucosal inflammation and mucus hypersecretion. Inhaled β_2 agonists and anti-cholinergic agents should be used routinely in patients who are symptomatic. Steroids, inhaled or oral, are a contentious issue: long-term oral steroids should be avoided because of their side-effects, especially in an elderly population. They are often used to treat exacerbations but with variable true benefit. The greatest challenge is to identify patients who have airways obstruction due to airway inflammation that could be ameliorated by long-term inhaled steroid use.

Objective response to short course oral steroid may predict responders to inhaled steroid therapy. Clues that suggest patients with appreciable reversibility include spontaneously variable symptoms, nocturnal awaking, early morning chest tightness or evidence of atopy including a venous blood eosinophilia. Improvement in spirometry following nebulised bronchodilator therapy may be a pragmatic way to decide.

COMPLICATIONS

Recurrent infections

Viral or bacterial infections are more likely with the viscid poorly cleared mucus that many of these patients secrete. It is an important cause of morbidity and probably adds to bronchial damage. Vaccination against influenza annually and once against pneumococcal serotypes is effective.

Exacerbations

Many of these patients suffer periods of increased breathlessness. This may be due to bronchial infection when fever, purulent sputum and a peripheral blood leucocytosis are present and further lung damage may be occurring. Alternatively, bronchial inflammation may occur without clear evidence of infection. Other causes of breathlessness must not be forgotten: many have bullae which may rupture to cause a pneumothorax. Ischaemic heart disease is common and pulmonary oedema may supervene. These patients are at increased risk of pulmonary emboli which can be difficult to detect: they already have abnormal ventilation and abnormal perfusion.

Breathlessness

With increasing airways obstruction, gas trapping and lung hyper-expansion result which place the respiratory muscles at an increasing mechanical disadvantage. The work of breathing increases, thus increasing the subjective sensations of breathlessness.

Hypoxia

Airways obstruction and gas trapping lead to uneven ventilation of a damaged vascular bed. Pulmonary vascular bed loss occurs as a result of lung destruction due to emphysema. Additionally, areas of hypoxic vasoconstriction and occlusion due to higher alveolar pressures contribute further to disturbed perfusion. The resulting perfusion disturbance and ventilatory abnormalities result in mismatching. In general, as airways obstruction worsens so does hypoxia. At severe levels of obstruction with FEV_1 below 1l, inadequate ventilation especially at night causes gradual carbon dioxide retention.

Cor pulmonale

This is a clinical syndrome of peripheral fluid retention, including abdominal ascites with pulmonary arterial hypertension as a consequence of chronic hypoxic lung disease, usually COPD. It is incorrectly termed 'right heart failure' as measures of right ventricular performance in life show function at least as well as in normal subjects. The salt and fluid retention is a renal response to chronic hypoxia. Patients initially develop fluid retention during exacerbations when hypoxia worsens, later developing chronic peripheral oedema. Diuretics may help the fluid retention with oxygen therapy. The hypoxic oedematous patient is referred to as a 'blue bloater' in contradistinction to the patient with more normal arterial blood gas tensions maintained at the expense of high ventilation, known as a 'pink puffer'. Both types of patient have similar degrees of emphysema but differ in response of their respiratory drive to hypoxia. Many of these patients are polycythaemic, so consideration should also be given to venesection. Thromboembolism prophylaxis is essential as these patients are relatively immobile, especially in hospital, and have little respiratory reserve such that even a small embolus could be devastating.

MANAGEMENT

Smoking cessation must be the most important goal. It prevents further lung damage at least and may reduce respiratory infections. It also allows the provision of long-term domiciliary oxygen therapy when appropriate.

Airways obstruction can be minimised using bronchodilators ideally inhaled via an effectively used delivery device. Theophyllines should be considered as an additional or alternative agent. Inhaled steroids may be appropriate if the patient has demonstrated the likelihood of steroid-responsiveness.

Vaccination against influenza and a number of pneumococcal serotypes should be offered. Bacterial respiratory infections must be treated promptly.

Oxygen therapy

Acute exacerbations of COPD are often associated with further deterioration in hypoxaemia and sometimes worsening hypercapnia. The deterioration in oxygenation can usually be corrected with low flow supplementary oxygen administered continuously via nasal cannulae. The goal of such treatment is to individually titrate oxygenation either to a recent p_aO_2 of the patient breathing air or to between 6.6–7.0 kPa, S_pO_2 around 90–92%, representing the 'knee' of the oxygen dissociation curve. As for any other therapy, the effectiveness of treatment must be measured by arterial blood gas estimations, especially p_aO_2 and H$^+$ ion levels. Worsening respiratory acidosis associated with appropriate oxygen therapy should prompt consideration of additional ventilatory support, rather than reducing oxygen therapy in fear of losing the 'hypoxic drive to respiration'.

Long-term domiciliary oxygen treatment delivering flow rates around 0.5–2 lpm for COPD has a survival benefit as well as improving peripheral oedema, polycythaemia and pulmonary hypertension. Patients must be stable when measured as hypoxic breathing air (<7.3 kPa), have experienced episodes of peripheral oedema and be non-smokers. To accrue the survival benefit, they require to use the treatment for at least 15 hours a day. In practice treatment should be continued overnight and as long as possible during the day. The most efficient provision is with an oxygen concentrator. Oxygen cylinders are cumbersome, not without risk and are rapidly exhausted. However, small portable cylinders may allow continued activity.

Disability

Many patients become significantly disabled by the progressive breathlessness. Appropriate pharmacological therapy is clearly of partial benefit. A rehabilitation programme to provide additional support is also required. This should include the following:

- Education improves the knowledge held by the patient and their family.
- Dietetic advice may help the significant weight loss sometimes seen.
- Physiotherapy exercise programmes counteract inactivity with the associated wasting and dwindling of respiratory and limb muscle function.
- Knowledge of appropriate social security benefits is important.
- Appliances and other aids at home improve activities of daily living.

There is increasing evidence that support leads to improvements in 'coping' skills. These feelings of control improve patients' perceived quality of life and may ameliorate demands on medical resources.

OTHER CONDITIONS TO CONSIDER

Lifelong non-smokers may develop breathlessness and evidence of airways obstruction. They may rarely have emphysema. Other conditions to consider include asthma and lymphangioleiomyomatosis, if young and female.

Bronchiolitis obliterans is a rare small airways disease associated with air trapping on a chest radiograph and airflow limitation. It can be caused by drugs, associated with rheumatoid arthritis or follow toxic gas inhalation. Less commonly it is a manifestation of graft-versus-host disease following bone marrow transplantation or rejection in transplanted lungs. It has been confusingly linked with organising pneumonitis by a pathological, though clinically meaningless, acronym 'BOOP'!

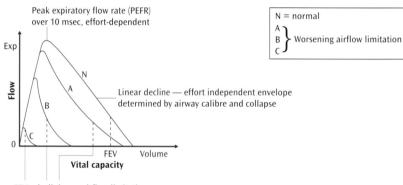

- FEV's declining as airflow limitation worsens
- Relative preservation of PEFR
- Early and increasing diminution of flow rates in mid expiration, the 'sag' in the down sloping expiration portion. This probably reflects small airways disease, the bronchiolitis of cigarette smokers
- Lack of variability in measures of airflow limitation or expired volumes reduces the value of frequent monitoring of PEFR rather than measuring FEV, for confirmation of diagnosis and severity or in contrast to asthma management

Fig. 1 **Flow volume curves in increasingly severe COPD.**

Case history 23

A 45-year-old fireman, a smoker only as a teenager, presents with progressive breathlessness over the last 9 months. He has airways obstruction on spirometry with a hyper-expanded chest clinically and radiologically.

Is this COPD?

COPD II

- The single most important management issue is to quit smoking.
- The early identification of individuals susceptible to the effects of cigarette smoke allows targeting of current anti-smoking strategies and may hold future therapeutic benefit.
- Early quitting is beneficial with increasing disability-free years.
- Long-term oxygen therapy for appropriately selected patients prolongs life.

LUNG CANCER I

EPIDEMIOLOGY

Although lung cancer is a malignancy of increasing age, with 70% of cases occurring in over 65-year-olds, it represents a significant socio-medical burden. In the developed world it has become the commonest cause of cancer death in men. In the UK it represents 1 in 3 cancer deaths and 25% of cancer registrations. In women it is the most rapidly rising cause of cancer mortality and is now second only to breast cancer. In Scotland it even exceeds breast cancer mortality, with lung cancer causing annually the loss of over 51 500 life-years compared with 21 000 life-years for breast cancer.

PATHOGENESIS

Tobacco

The great potential for primary prevention in lung cancer is self-evident. Around 90% of lung cancer is attributable to cigarette smoking. Rates in men in the developed countries are falling slightly concomitant with reductions in smoking: in contrast to those seen in women. The evidence implicating passive smoking in the genesis of lung tumours is not as robust. Very few patients (< 10%) are true 'never smokers'.

Tobacco smoke contains over 40 different oxidants and carcinogens, including benzpyrenes, acrolein and benzene. In susceptible patients these cause neoplastic change at the bronchial epithelium. Despite exposure of the whole mucosa to inhaled compounds, the development of tumours is usually focal. The activation of tumour promoting genes and inhibition of tumour suppressor genes (including p53, see box) occurs. Depending on the host's immunological response, cell reproduction may continue with this loss of normal cellular growth and differentiation mechanisms. This results in a macroscopic tumour (Fig. 1). Hence, the substantial rise in lung cancer that we are still seeing reflects the widespread uptake of cigarette smoking earlier in the last century. Even a complete cessation now of smoking would take many years to see an effect on lung cancer.

That only 20% of cigarette smokers develop lung cancer demonstrates the role of inter-individual factors that include:

- **Genetics.** Non-smokers with a family history of lung cancer are at greater risk compared to non-smokers without a pedigree.
- **Environment.** Rural populations usually have lower incidence rates than urban communities.
- **Social deprivation.** Communities scoring highly for social deprivation show higher rates than less deprived areas, even when corrected for cigarette consumption. Deprivation may be a surrogate for factors such as dietary intake of antioxidant vitamins and minerals.

Other causes

Asbestos is an inert natural rock silicate with uses in industry. Unfortunately, it is also a carcinogen in its own right. The risk of exposure to asbestos is synergistic with tobacco smoke. To a non-smoker the risk of lung cancer from asbestos exposure is five times that of an unexposed non-smoker, while in a smoking worker the exposure risk is 55 times that of an unexposed non-smoker. Other occupational causes of lung cancer include the inhalation of radioactive gases, including environmental exposure to radon, and workplace chemicals that include

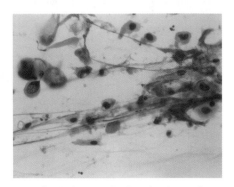

Fig. 2 **Cytological examination of early morning sputum with malignant (orange and green staining) squamous cells.** (Image courtesy of Dr G. Rebello.)

arsenic, chromate and those of the electronics industries.

CLINICAL PRESENTATION

Clinical presentation is usually late in the tumour's natural history. Furthermore, co-morbidity in an aged and largely uncomplaining group of patients contributes to the poor survival rates. Overall, a mere 8% of diagnosed patients will survive 5 years, a rate that has changed little in the past three decades. The current poor outlook for patients with this disease might be improved by a high index of clinical suspicion for earlier diagnosis to offer more patients potentially curative surgery. Barely 20% of patients at presentation have disease sufficiently localised for attempts at curative surgery.

SCREENING

The combination of a readily identifiable population at increased risk of developing lung cancer and such poor survival due in part to late presentation would suggest a need for screening programmes. However, programmes utilising chest radiography and sputum cytology in a number of healthcare systems around the world have been disappointing. There has been no objective evidence of a survival benefit in any of these screened populations.

CLASSIFICATION

Clinically and pathologically, it is useful to consider malignant lung tumours as either small (undifferentiated) cell lung cancer (SCLC, about 20% of lung can-

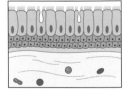
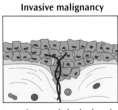

Molecular changes	Carcinoma in situ	Invasive malignancy
Activation of tumour promoting genes	Host immune response	Invasion and desimination
Inactivation of suppressor genes	Continued cell division and loss of differentiation	
Growth factors enhancing	New blood vessel strands	

Fig. 1 **The development of lung cancer.**

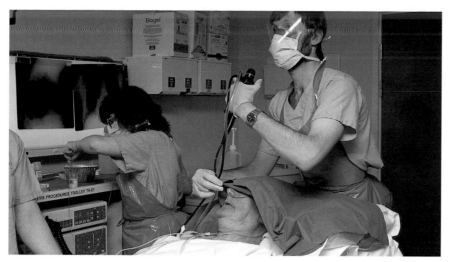

Fig. 3 **Flexible bronchoscopy.**

cers) or non-small cell lung cancer (NSCLC).

SCLC

This can be diagnosed with a high degree of confidence, even cytologically. It typically presents as a bulky central lung tumour with early spread to mediastinum and to extrathoracic sites. The tumour cells proliferate rapidly and untreated patients have a median survival of a mere 3–4 months from presentation.

NSCLC

NSCLC covers a heterogeneous group. Pathologists recognise:

- squamous cell carcinomas (now about 20–25%)
- adenocarcinoma (40%)
- undifferentiated (non-small cell) carcinomas
- truly mixed tumours.

These tumours may be more difficult to type with confidence on cytology or small biopsy specimens, hence the usefulness of NSCLC as a classification. Adenocarcinomas have increased in frequency over the last 2–3 decades. In recent US and UK studies outside ethnic Chinese populations, adenocarcinoma is now the most common form of NSCLC. SCLC is also increasing as a proportion of all lung cancer. These changes may reflect the increase in women smokers and changes in the type and burning qualities of current tobacco.

PATHOLOGICAL DIAGNOSIS

The majority of patients need the clinical or radiological suspicion of lung cancer to be pathologically confirmed. There is always a balance between what is possible and what is therapeutically appropri-

ate for an individual patient. Techniques available include:

- Cytological examination of early morning sputum (Fig. 2). This may be more readily obtainable and is less invasive than bronchoscopy for central airway disease. Three adequate samples on consecutive mornings should be considered standard.
- Flexible bronchoscopy for central endobronchial (Fig. 3) or peribronchial disease. Secretions can be aspirated and washings, needle aspiration or brushings obtained for cytology with mucosal biopsies for pathology. A partial assessment of the suitability of the patient for surgery can also be made.
- Pleural aspiration and biopsy in the presence of pleural fluid and hence possible pleural deposits of tumour.
- Needle aspiration of neck nodes for cytology.
- Transthoracic needle aspiration or biopsy of subpleural masses (Fig. 4).
- Thoracoscopy and biopsy of pleural, mediastinal or subpleural pulmonary masses.
- Liver or bone biopsy of possible deposits.

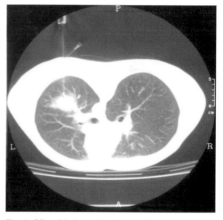

Fig. 4 **CT guided needle biopsy of lung mass.**

p53 and cigarette smoke

The human gene called p53 is a tumour suppressor gene that initiates programmed cell death in malignant cells. Specific point mutations in p53 preventing cell death are common in human cancers, particularly lung tumours. Tobacco smoke contains a carcinogen benzo[a]pyrene, a metabolite of which has been demonstrated to cause at least one of these specific mutational changes to p53 gene in a number of experimental cell types. There may well be other carcinogens which produce specific mutations in this or other tumour suppressor genes. This provides the first molecular evidence directly linking cigarette smoke with the genesis of lung cancer. Control of such gene activity may be an avenue for future anti-tumour therapies.

Case history 24

A 50-year-old man presents with pain in his left hip of gradual onset over days. He has a central mass on his chest radiograph.

- How would you confirm your suspicion of lung cancer?
- Why does he have bone pain?
- Blood results demonstrate Na:122; Ca: 2.6; alb 34; alk phosphate: 650. Why?

Lung cancer I

- Lung cancer is the most common solid tumour affecting males in western Europe.
- Tobacco smoking is the major and most easily preventable, but not the sole, risk factor.
- Clinical presentation is often late; the diagnosis may not be readily apparent, a factor contributing to poor survival rates over the last three decades.

LUNG CANCER II

CLINICAL FEATURES

Less than 10% of patients are asymptomatic at presentation. These cases are often discovered as a result of a chest radiograph performed for another reason and usually present as a solitary peripheral lesion (SPL). An SPL may be benign or malignant, primary or secondary (Fig. 1). Benign disease, especially tuberculo-

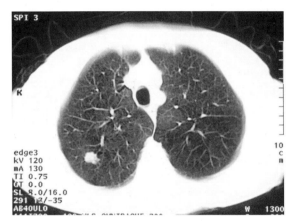

Fig. 1 **Solitary peripheral lesion.**

sis granulomas or benign tumours, should always be considered. There are no radiological features absolutely characteristic of benignity, but the presence of certain patterns of calcification, occurrence at the site of known benign disease and previous radiology demonstrating slow if any change in size are all helpful.

An SPL is more likely to be malignant with increasing age of the patient, particularly if a smoker. If there is a known primary tumour elsewhere, or there is clinical evidence of one, the SPL is likely to be a secondary. If the available evidence suggests a primary and the patient is fit, then curative resection should be planned. This will provide histological

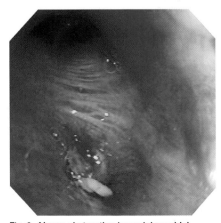

Fig. 2 **Airway obstruction by endobronchial tumour.**

confirmation and potential cure at the same time. Such a policy accepts finite resection rates both for lesions that turn out to be benign (less than 5% and usually tuberculosis), and for those that with the passage of time become evident as secondaries (up to 10% of adenocarcinomas).

Primary tumours

Of the remaining presentations, one-third have symptoms due to the primary tumour. New cough or change in a long-standing cough, even without haemoptysis, is an important symptom in a smoker, even if a chest radiograph is normal. The consequences of large airway obstruction (Fig. 2) that may include inspiratory stridor, 'slow to radiologically resolve' pneumonia, undue or worsening breathlessness that may be difficult to distinguish from the many other causes.

Metastases

A further third of presentations are due to intrathoracic (Fig. 3) or extrathoracic (Fig. 4) metastases.

Systemic symptoms

The remaining patients present due to systemic symptoms. Weight loss may result from cytokines secreted by the tumour. Lassitude is also characteristic.

Non-metastatic or para-neoplastic manifestations arise by the production of circulating factors derived from the primary tumour, and may be apparent at initial presentation or later. Treatment of the primary may not always alleviate these manifestations. The common patterns are:

- Bone:
  —clubbing, rarely in SCLC
  —hypertrophic pulmonary osteoarthropathy, painful wrists and ankles from new bone formation, usually squamous or adenocarcinoma.

- Endocrine:
  —ADH secretion, usually by SCLC causing hyponatraemia the commonest electrolyte upset; patients become confused, require fluid restriction and demeclocycline
  —non-metastatic hypercalcaemia, due to PTH-like substances secreted usually by squamous tumours
  —Cushing's syndrome: rapid onset with weakness (myopathy and hypokalaemia) and hyperglycaemia from ectopic ACTH secretion.

- Haematology: coagulopathy,

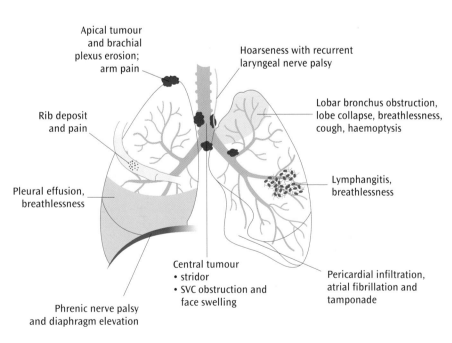

Fig. 3 **Intrathoracic spread of lung cancer with associated symptoms.**

Apical tumour and brachial plexus erosion; arm pain

Hoarseness with recurrent laryngeal nerve palsy

Lobar bronchus obstruction, lobe collapse, breathlessness, cough, haemoptysis

Rib deposit and pain

Lymphangitis, breathlessness

Pleural effusion, breathlessness

Central tumour
• stridor
• SVC obstruction and face swelling

Pericardial infiltration, atrial fibrillation and tamponade

Phrenic nerve palsy and diaphragm elevation

disseminated intravascular coagulation with a consumptive bleeding disorder or venous thromboses and superficial phlebitis.

- Neurology: rare syndromes in a spectrum from peripheral neuropathy through myaesthenia to dermatomyositis.

MANAGEMENT

Surgery

Surgery for NSCLC, and probably for very early SCLC, still offers the best chance of cure, with a 5-year survival of 50% in early stage NSCLC. This requires a thorough clinical, laboratory and radiological assessment to ensure the patient is fit to withstand single-lung anaesthesia and major surgery, along with an absence of metastatic malignant disease outwith the planned resection of lobe or lung. This usually requires:

- Pulmonary function to include FEV_1 FVC, Kco, walking distance, resting electrocardiogram. Cardiac reserve may have to be assessed further with either an exercise treadmill test or coronary angiography.
- Biochemistry including calcium and liver enzymes.
- Plain radiology of chest.
- CT scan of chest particularly to identify mediastinal glands that

should be sampled for histology. Many centres include CT of liver but ultrasound is at least as good as CT and liver deposits are unlikely in the absence of an elevated alkaline phosphatase.

Thoracic surgical teams will formally explore the mediastinum to sample nodes directed by the CT scan before undertaking formal resection.

Alternative therapies

Surgical cure should be the goal in fit patients with resectable NSCLC. In patients with resectable disease, but who decline surgery or have intercurrent (usually cardiac) disease, radical radiotherapy may be an option with cure rates not that different from surgery. SCLC can be treated with cyclical combination chemotherapy, providing a median survival of around 12 months with an increased quality of life.

Palliative care

Palliative care, in the broadest multidisciplinary sense, should begin at diagnosis and the breaking of that bad news to the patient. Radiotherapy can palliate the symptoms of bone pain, significant haemoptysis, breathlessness from lobe or lung collapse consequent on airway obstruction or impending collapse, superior mediastinal obstruction and spinal

cord compression. Radiotherapy offers little for the non-specific symptoms of lassitude and weight loss. New chemotherapy regimes even for inoperable NSCLC may help such symptoms. Control by pharmacological or non-pharmacological means of pain, cough and breathlessness in particular are important. Metabolic disturbances including hyponatraemia and hypercalcaemia can present insidiously, and should be actively sought. These will respond to appropriate therapy. Teflon injection of a paralysed vocal cord under local anaesthetic can help voice quality. As survival is in general poor, the quality of life should be paramount in the management of such patients.

Future therapies

Advancements in understanding tumour development and cell biology will allow a multi-faceted approach to lung cancer

---

Case history 25

A 50-year-old man has a bone secondary from lung cancer. Blood results demonstrate: calcium 2–7 mmol/l, albumin 34 g/l, alkaline phosphatase 650 u.

What treatment could you offer?

Lung cancer II

- The most useful clinico-pathological classification is into SCLC and NSCLC.
- SCLC is an aggressive central tumour with a median survival of 3 months untreated.
- For many patients, symptom control is the main therapeutic goal.

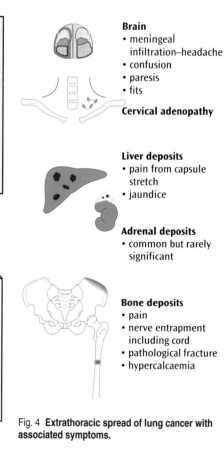

Brain
- meningeal infiltration–headache
- confusion
- paresis
- fits

Cervical adenopathy

Liver deposits
- pain from capsule stretch
- jaundice

Adrenal deposits
- common but rarely significant

Bone deposits
- pain
- nerve entrapment including cord
- pathological fracture
- hypercalcaemia

Fig. 4 **Extrathoracic spread of lung cancer with associated symptoms.**

Table 1 **Quality of life – symptom-relieving strategies in lung cancer**

Breathlessness
Identify and treat conventionally heart failure, COPD, anaemia, etc
Pleural effusion
•   drain and pleurodese
Lobar or main stem obstruction
•   radiotherapy
endoluminal tumour
ablation
•   tracheobronchial stent
Lymphangitis
•   steroid trial
Radiation pneumonitis
•   steroid trial
'Tumour associated'
•   breathing relaxation techniques
•   pacing activities
•   other non-pharmacological techniques such as aromatherapy and acupuncture
•   liquid morphine
•   nebulised morphine
•   anxiolytic
Haemoptysis
Radiotherapy
•   external beam
•   intraluminal (brachytherapy)
Endobrachial cautery argon plasma
Pain
Bone pain
•   non-steroidal analgesic and opiate
•   radiotherapy
Neural pain
•   steroid
•   anticonvulsant, e.g. gabapentin
Anorexia, weight loss
•   small frequent meal
•   increase spice/herb use
•   steroid
•   anti-inflammatory drug
Cough
Oral opiate
Nebulised lignocaine (with care)

METASTATIC SPREAD AND THE LUNG

METASTATIC SPREAD AND THE LUNG

HAEMATOGENOUS SPREAD

The lung, in receiving all of the cardiac output, is a common site for haematogenous tumour deposition, even secondary spread from a lung primary. Other common primary sites include gut (stomach, rectal), genitourinary, breast and malignant melanoma (Fig. 1). Pulmonary deposits may be asymptomatic or appear before the primary is clinically apparent. Such haematogenous secondaries appear as discrete 'cannon-ball' masses enlarging on chest radiographs over time (Fig. 2). They tend to be subpleural and lower zone. When small, secondaries need differentiation from benign granulomas on CT scanning. An isolated metastasis requires differentiation from a primary lung tumour. A solitary secondary may be considered for metastectomy either for relief of symptoms or as a debulking procedure. There may be a worthwhile time delay before further secondaries develop. Any other treatment must be governed by the primary tumour.

PLEURAL DEPOSITS

Pleural tumour deposits present as pleural effusions, rarely as discrete pleural masses. Investigation by Abrams biopsy or thoracoscopy should confirm the diagnosis. Stomach, breast and ovarian tumours often spread to the pleura, with therapeutic gain in discovering primary tumours in the latter two sites (see pp. 66–67).

INTERSTITIAL LYMPHATIC SPREAD

Lymphangitis carcinomatosis has a suggestive radiological pattern of progressive interstitial shadowing, including septal and intrapulmonary (Kerley A) lymphatic lines (Fig. 3). The clinical picture is of a patient, usually with a known primary, complaining of relentless breathlessness. Their distress is often seemingly out of proportion to the apparent plain X-ray abnormalities, but reflects the increasingly stiff lungs held rigid by a lattice-work of tumour within the lymphatics. If performed, CT scanning will demonstrate nodules of tumour along a pattern of distended lymphatics.

ENDOBRONCHIAL SECONDARIES

These metastases that occur on the luminal side of the bronchi are rare. Those that occur in the central airways and, hence, are visible at bronchoscopy represent about 1 per 150 bronchoscopies for cancer (Fig. 4).

Most are found as an explanation for haemoptysis or obstructing symptoms. Often there is a past history of the primary cancer; colon and breast are the most common (Fig. 5).

RARE TUMOURS

Bronchioloalveolar cell carcinoma

This is a form of adenocarcinoma that has a propensity for spread along the alveolar walls and into lymphatics. Insidious breathlessness, a cough productive of frothy sputum and a progressive pneumonia-like illness are usual presentations. Chest radiology demonstrates alveolar shadowing (Fig. 6). Cytology of sputum or bronchoscopic washings will confirm malignancy and bronchoscopic lung biopsy may demonstrate the characteristic pattern of alveolar wall spread. Often at diagnosis

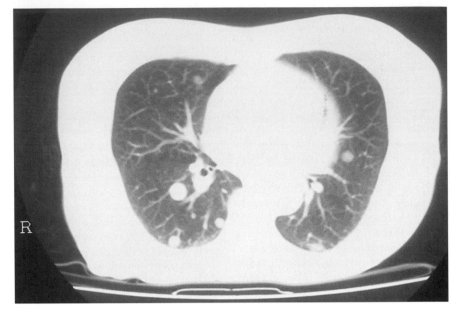

Fig. 2 **Multiple, mainly peripheral and variable in size — these are the characteristic features of multiple blood-borne lung metastases.**

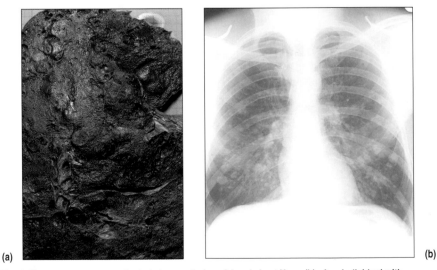

(a)   (b)

Fig. 1 **Haematogenous spread: whole lung pathology (a) and chest X-ray (b) of an individual with malignant melanoma metastases in the lung.**

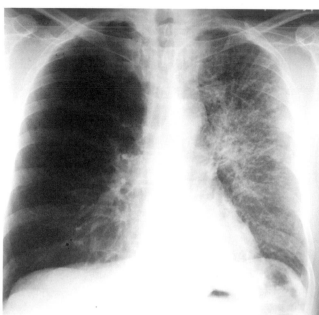

Fig. 3 **Interstitial lymphatic spread: chest X-ray.**

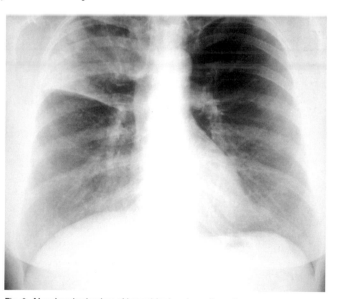

Fig. 5 **Metastatic spread to the lungs – common primary sites.**

(Figure labels from Fig. 5:)

Haematogenous spread
Large deposits (e.g. from renal, melanoma)
Miliary small deposits (e.g. from thyroid carcinoma)

Endobronchial deposits
• colon
• breast

Pleural deposits
(often with fluid)
• adenocarcinoma
• breast
• ovary
• gut
• lung

Lymphangitic spread

contralateral lung is involved preventing attempts at curative surgery. Chemotherapy is of limited benefit. The distressing symptoms of cough and breathlessness need palliation.

Bronchial carcinoid

This is the commonest benign lung tumour. Embryologically it is derived from fore-gut neuroendocrine cells. It very rarely presents as the carcinoid syndrome of flushing and diarrhoea (in contrast to mid gut carcinoid tumours with hepatic metastases). Biologically, there is a spectrum of behaviours.

The 'typical' carcinoid tumours are vascular endobronchial polypoid tumours that present usually in young women as either recurrent haemoptysis or recurrent infections with radiological infiltrates distal to bronchial obstruction. Sleeve resection of the bronchial wall with the tumour should be curative.

Histologically, 'atypical carcinoids' may present as above but tend to behave more as malignant tumours with local and distant spread. They are chemosensitive. There is some morphological and embryological basis in considering a spectrum of behaviour from typical carcinoid through 'atypical' to small cell lung tumours.

Lymphangioleiomyomatosis (LAM)

This is a malignancy of immature pulmonary smooth muscle cells and is believed to originate from the lymphatics. Infiltration of bronchioles leads to focal emphysema and air trapping. Veno-occlusion and lymphatic involvement contributes to the clinical picture. It occurs almost exclusively in women of reproductive age, and growth seems dependent on oestrogen hormones.

Presentation is in early to middle adult life with breathlessness and airflow limitation. Frequent complications include haemoptysis, pneumothorax or chylous effusions. The chest radiograph will show a reticular pattern to the lung parenchyma. High-resolution CT lung scanning will demonstrate thin-walled cystic airspaces. Treatment is supportive with progesterone until a menopause.

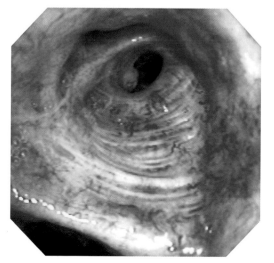

Fig. 4 **Endobronchial deposit.** This lady presented with haempotysis and a normal chest radiograph. Biopsy confirmed mucin-secreting adenocarcinoma, histologically similar to colonic cancer removed 4 years previously.

Fig. 6 **Alveolar shadowing of bronchioalveolar cell carcinoma.**

Metastatic spread and the lung

• The lung and pleura are common sites for metastatic tumour deposition.

PULMONARY THROMBOEMBOLI

Intravascular thrombi originate in systemic veins, usually in the deep veins of the lower limb, and migrate into the pulmonary circulation. They are relatively frequent within hospitalised patients, can be difficult to diagnose and yet fatal. Several studies have demonstrated prevalences in a hospitalised population of venous clot ranging from less than 10% when associated with minor medical illness to exceeding 70% following surgery for traumatic hip fractures. Embolism into the pulmonary circulation may cause 10% of all hospital deaths.

MECHANISMS

Intravascular thrombus formation usually starts in the deep venous system of the calf. This is called a 'deep vein thrombosis' (DVT). The mechanisms that prevent the formation and propagation of intravascular thrombus fail as a result of:

- Abnormal or damaged vascular endothelium, especially important for arterial thrombosis and within grafts, less of a factor in calf veins except in recurrent venous thrombosis.
- Blood stasis or pooling, usually resulting from immobility. Immobility is the most prevalent predisposing factor, closely followed by the cause of the immobility. Trauma, following surgery, and many medical illnesses are associated with an acute inflammatory response that leads to the following.
- Imbalance between the blood's procoagulant and thrombolytic properties that favours coagulation. Conditions include malignancy, particularly disseminated adenocarcinomas, therapy with oestrogens either as contraceptives or hormone replacement, or the antiphospholipid antibody syndrome. Moreover rare inherited deficiencies of particular fibrinolytic proteins can favour a procoagulant tendency.

DEEP CALF VEIN THROMBOSIS

Often such clot is clinically silent though localised calf discomfort, swelling and warmth may occur. Such features are not diagnostic but are more likely when clot propogates proximally into the thigh veins. It is this proximal extension that is most at risk of embolising. The presence of clot should be actively confirmed or excluded by radiological investigation.

The two most available imaging investigations are:

- **Lower limb ascending venography.** This is considered to be the gold standard investigation. The technique uses intravenous contrast to radiologically outline the deep venous system of the legs from calf extending proximally into femoral and iliac vessels. Thrombus is demonstrated as consistent filling defects within the outlined vessels. The technique involves radiation exposure and the slight risk of reaction to the radio-opaque contrast used.
- **Doppler ultrasound examination of the veins.** This utilises the demonstration of a Doppler signal by flowing blood with the deep veins. The absence of a spontaneous flow signal in non-compressible veins can be taken as evidence of occlusive thrombus. Although it is less sensitive than venography in imaging the calf veins, it is as good from popliteal to iliac vessels. Being free of ionising radiation, such examinations can readily be repeated if clinical circumstances require.

Deep venous clot proximal to the calf is treated with anticoagulant therapy to prevent further extension, traditionally heparin alone or followed by warfarin. During such therapy the existing clot will be lysed by endogenous systems. This recanalisation is at the expense of losing the competence of venous valves. The long term sequelae of such venous incompetence includes the 'post-phlebitic' leg with chronic swelling, pain and ulceration. There is some evidence that treatment by thrombolysis (rather than anticoagulant therapy) and long-term wearing of support hosiery may reduce this complication.

PULMONARY EMBOLI (PE)

Proximal leg vein thrombus may break off and travel through the right heart with the potential there for outflow obstruction, before lodging and occluding part of the pulmonary vascular bed. The consequences of such acute embolisation are:

- Breathlessness due to the loss of pulmonary vascular bed but without the degree of localised circulatory compromise that results in lung infarction. There may be few clinical signs.
- Pulmonary infarction syndrome with sudden onset pleurisy and cough often productive of blood with undue breathlessness. Clinical signs may include localised crackles, pleural fluid and occasionally a pleural rub. Chest radiographs may show the development of intrapulmonary pleural-based shadowing with pleural fluid.
- Sudden collapse as a result of substantial clot causing obstruction to the outflow tract of the right ventricle or a major pulmonary artery. The symptoms may not be immediately recognised for what they represent: acute central chest pain, breathlessness and circulatory collapse, systemic hypotension but with distended neck veins: a 'right heart syndrome'. Death may ensue. Substantial loss of the pulmonary vascular bed occurs but the cardiovascular effects are more than the mere consequences of vascular bed loss. Right ventricular and even left ventricular dysfunction with the release of vasoactive inflammatory mediators as a result of the intravascular clot is as important. In contrast, closing the vascular supply to one lung surgically, or by vessel occlusion with inert material, causes only transient haemodynamic effects.

Repeated embolisation of clot to the pulmonary circulation over days to weeks can lead to the syndrome of 'cor pulmonale' with breathlessness, hypoxia, right heart strain and fluid retention.

Clinical features

The clinical features of pulmonary embolism are non-specific. There are few other potentially lethal conditions for which our clinical diagnostic accuracy is so poor. In an acutely ill or post-operative patient there are a number of other diagnostic possibilities, including pneumonia. The entire clinical picture including an assessment of risk supplemented by chest radiography, electrocardiography and arterial blood gases can provide a feel for the likelihood of a pulmonary embolus or the possibility of an alternate diagnosis. Further investigation has to be performed to confirm or refute the diagnosis of pulmonary emboli because of the potential lethality and the therapeutic implications.

Further investigation can be directed to either confirming the presence of deep leg vein clot from which embolisation was possible, or confirming pulmonary embolisation.

The pulmonary arterial circulation can be imaged at pulmonary angiography where clot can be visualised as filling defects (Fig. 1). This is the probably the definitive investigation but is not always available. Isotope lung scanning provides a simpler means to image lung perfusion (Fig. 2) but interpretation of such scans is not always easy and over-interpretation is a risk. About 60% of lung scans are unhelpful in either confirming or refuting pulmonary embolism as the diagnosis. In such cases additional imaging is required which may include leg vein imaging. Echocardiography is often readily available, can demonstrate acute right heart strain with pulmonary hypertension and helps to exclude other causes of an acute right heart syndrome. Alternative techniques include helical CT scanning with contrast (p. 77) and magnetic resonance imaging; both techniques may be useful in demonstrating large pulmonary vessel clot.

Management

Anticoagulant therapy is the mainstay of treatment. It should be commenced once the diagnosis is suspected, as long as there are no contraindications to such therapy. Once anticoagulant therapy is commenced, mortality falls to less than 10%. Unfortunately, only 10% of deaths attributed to PE received any such treatment prior to death.

Anticoagulant therapy should be commenced as heparin, and warfarin is then started. Heparin can be discontinued once the effect of warfarin is therapeutic. Heparin alone is used in the later stages of pregnancy, but with the added risks of immune thrombocytopenia and of osteoporosis with such long-term therapy.

Recurrent embolisation that continues

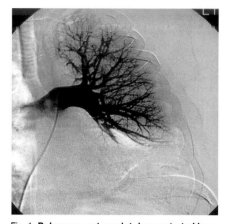

Fig. 1 **Pulmonary artery clot demonstrated by contrast angiogram.**

from leg vein clot once anticoagulation is established requires consideration of an inferior vena caval interruption device. This is usually a 'caval filter', an umbrella net that is placed percutaneously and acts truly as a filter.

The role of thrombolysis in acute massive PE associated with major haemodynamic upset is still controversial but may be lifesaving.

The most efficient way to prevent both fatal and non-fatal pulmonary emboli and DVT is aggressive prophylaxis in at-risk hospital patients. This can be achieved using mechanical techniques including early mobilisation and leg compression devices. Subcutaneous heparin as the low molecular weight heparins now available are effective and simple to use. No technique is completely reliable in preventing pulmonary emboli.

Miscellaneous sources of thrombotic pulmonary emboli

These are summarised in Figure 3. There are rare sources of pulmonary emboli that should be considered in any of the pulmonary thromboembolism syndromes when leg vein clot is demonstrably absent. These include:

- Clot from the right heart including mural thrombus in dilated right

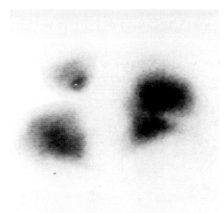

Fig. 2 **Isotope perfusion lung scan illustrating impaired delivery to left upper and right lower lung regions.** These perfusion defects represent vascular bed obstruction from emboli (chest radiograph normal).

ventricles.
- Embolisation from the renal veins can occur. The material is either tumour spreading directly along the renal vein or renal vein thrombosis especially in amyloidosis.
- Right heart myxomas are exceptionally rare.

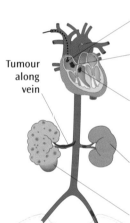

Thrombus, often infected on central venous catheter

Right axial myxoma

Right ventricular mural thrombus, following infarction or when dilated and poorly functioning

Amyloid kidney, renal vein thrombosis

Renal carcinoma with tumour extension along or in situ thrombosis

Tumour along vein

Pelvic vein clot

Fig. 3 **Miscellaneous sources of thrombotic pulmonary emboli.**

Case history 26

A 30-year-old female on the oral contraceptive pill with a history of poorly controlled asthma presents with rapid onset severe breathlessness and pleurisy. A chest radiograph is normal. Having started treatment for pulmonary emboli, how could you confirm your suspicions?

Pulmonary thromboemboli

- Pulmonary embolisation is potentially lethal and often complicates hospitalisation and major illness.
- It can be difficult to diagnose, with patients receiving risky therapy when they have not suffered the condition and other patients going untreated for an undiagnosed life-threatening condition.
- Clinical assessment alone is insufficient for diagnosis or upon which to base long-term treatment decisions. Radiological imaging is essential to confirm the diagnosis.
- Preventative therapy, whether physical or pharmacological, is the most cost-effective.

NON-THROMBOTIC PULMONARY EMBOLI/HYPERTENSION/MALFORMATIONS

In addition to intravascular thrombus, the pulmonary vascular bed can filter a range of other embolising materials.

Gas emboli

Usually the gas is air entering the vascular system during cannulation of central veins with inadequate head-down tilt or following chest trauma. Underwater divers ascending too quickly may create systemic venous nitrogen bubbles which can also be filtered by the lungs. The consequences depend on the volume of the gas. It may be clinically silent, pulmonary infarction may occur or embolisation into the systemic circulation if there is a patent right-to-left shunt. Large gas volumes may froth within the beating right atrium and cause acute right heart obstruction which is rapidly fatal.

Fat emboli

Long bone fractures or the orthopaedic reaming of the marrow space for intramedullary nailing will release fat globules from the bone marrow into the systemic venous circulation. Many are filtered by the lungs. However, there is often evidence of systemic embolisation in the absence of an overt right-to-left shunt. This is due perhaps to a temporary increase in right atrial pressure transiently restoring patency to an atrial septal defect thus allowing easily deformable fat to pass through.

There is a range of clinical effects as acute lung injury develops. Mild hypoxia may be discovered only by measuring arterial blood gases or transcutaneous oxygen saturation. Conversely, severe respiratory distress may develop with mental confusion and petechiae over the skin of the upper trunk, reflecting systemic capillary embolisation. Management is supportive. Although the diagnosis is often suspected clinically, it may be confirmed by microscopy of urine, sputum or pulmonary capillary blood (if a pulmonary artery flotation catheter is sited) looking for fat globules.

Septic emboli

With septic emboli, most patients are unwell with systemic upset and features of pulmonary infarction or infection with fever, cough and purulent sputum and pleurisy. The sources of embolisation include infected indwelling central venous catheters or the right heart structures. Such venous catheters have usually been used long-term for nutrition or drug therapy. Occasionally, recently inserted catheters become coated with thrombus that becomes infected.

Infective right heart endocarditis is rare outwith indwelling central venous catheters or intravenous drug misuse. The micro-organism may cause an aggressive sepsis with rapid valve destruction or a more indolent course.

Tumour emboli

Much metastatic spread into the lungs is haematogenous. Renal carcinomas especially propagate along the renal veins into the inferior vena cava where embolisation to the lungs may occur.

Amniotic fluid embolisation

This is a rare but potentially devastating complication of childbirth. The mother collapses in respiratory distress during labour and management is supportive. The differential diagnosis includes massive pulmonary emboli or haemorrhage.

PULMONARY HYPERTENSION

Pulmonary arterial hypertension occurs when systolic pressures exceed 20/ at rest or 30/ upon exercise. This usually occurs as a result of a cardiac output being ejected into a pulmonary vascular bed with an abnormal vascular resistance due to:

- occlusion by emboli or in situ thrombosis
- narrowing due to hypoxia-induced vasoconstriction (the pulmonary vascular response to hypoxia), permanent structural changes consequent on a chronically hyperdynamic circulation or vessel inflammation in vasculitis with in situ thrombosis
- destruction as in emphysema.

Elevated blood viscosity alone may rarely increase pulmonary vascular pressures. Elevated pulmonary arterial pressures may also occur secondary to pulmonary venous hypertension consequent on left ventricular dysfunction or a structural abnormality such as mitral valve stenosis.

Pulmonary hypertension most commonly accompanies chronic hypoxic lung disease, especially COPD. The combination of chronic hypoxia-induced vasoconstriction, subsequent structural changes within the vessel walls and the vascular bed destruction accompanying emphysema results in an elevated pulmonary vascular resistance.

Causes

- **Chronic hypoxic lung disease.** Pulmonary arterial hypertension is most commonly the consequence of chronic hypoxic lung disease, especially COPD. Occasionally, bronchiectasis, pulmonary fibrosis and cystic fibrosis may be the primary lung diseases.
- **Thromboemboli.** Chronic recurrent pulmonary emboli should be considered. Pleurisy may not be a prominent symptom, but increasing breathlessness is invariably present and is sometimes stepwise in its deterioration. The clinical signs of pulmonary hypertension may be subtle and lung signs may be absent. Chest radiographs may demonstrate flitting intrapulmonary and pleural shadowing. An isotope lung perfusion scan, with a ventilation scan if a chest radiograph is abnormal, should be diagnostic.
- **Vascular bed closure.** Pulmonary vasculitis should be suspected (especially in the context of sero-positive rheumatoid arthritis or systemic sclerosis) when the signs of pulmonary hypertension and estimated pulmonary arterial pressures are out of proportion to the known parenchymal lung disease and hypoxaemia. In parts of the developing world visceral larval migrans of schistosomiasis causes pulmonary bed occlusion and hypertension. Other rare causes include idiosyncratic drug reactions, the most notorious being slimming agents such as aminorex in the 1970s and more recently the 'fluramines'. Patent cardiac defects with left-to-right shunting result in a hyperdynamic pulmonary circulation that causes secondary vascular changes
- **Primary pulmonary hypertension.** Patients present with progressive breathlessness and the clinical features of pulmonary arterial hypertension in the absence of any apparent cause. The most important secondary causes to exclude are recurrent pulmonary emboli and structural heart abnormalities. The vascular abnormality is a combination of

vasoconstriction and structural changes within the walls of the small arteries. It is rare but commoner in women and the diagnosis is often delayed, sometimes by many years. With the ready availability now of Doppler echocardiography the diagnosis is easier to confirm.

Clinical features

These are often discovered in the context of COPD, but when occurring in isolation as in primary pulmonary hypertension the signs are often missed. Progressive breathlessness is usual, sometimes with vague central chest discomfort due to myocardial ischaemia. Palpation of the precordium demonstrates a parasternal heave of right ventricular hypertrophy. Upon auscultation a prominent pulmonary component of the second heart sound will be heard and may be palpable. Acute elevations of pulmonary arterial pressures may cause right ventricular dilatation, subsequent tricuspid valve incompetence, a tender expansile liver, ascites and peripheral oedema.

The electrocardiograph (Fig. 1) may show peaked p waves of right atrial hypertrophy and features of right ventricular dominance that include partial or complete right bundle branch block and right axis shift. A chest radiograph often demonstrates prominent and enlarged pulmonary arteries at the hilar, though determining the structures contributing to the hilar shadows sometimes can be difficult. Radiographic features of any underlying lung disease such as emphysema may be apparent.

Measurement

Colour Doppler echocardiography in the presence of even trivial tricuspid valve regurgitation can non-invasively estimate pulmonary artery pressure as right ventricular systolic pressure.

Direct measurement by invasive right heart catheterisation and pulmonary artery catheterisation is rarely required in routine clinical practice. The procedure can be diagnostic in the presence of a left-to-right intracardiac shunt, such as a patent atrial septal defect. Detailed blood sampling within the cardiac chamber should demonstrate a step up in measured oxygen saturations at the level of the shunt (Fig. 2).

Therapy

Aggressive treatment of the underlying condition is important. Relief of hypoxia by long-term oxygen therapy and prompt treatment of infections is necessary. Currently available vasodilators are of little benefit. Lung transplantation is the only definitive treatment.

PULMONARY ARTERIOVENOUS MALFORMATIONS

These are rare vascular channels that directly link a pulmonary arterial branch with a vein. They develop either as an isolated abnormality or in the context of systemic disease, especially hereditary haemorrhagic telangiectasia or chronic liver disease as the hepato-pulmonary syndrome.

Although often asymptomatic, they are sometimes associated with systemic hypoxaemia. More important as a consequence of the right-to-left intrapulmonary vascular shunt is the appreciable life-time risk of systemic embolisation. This can produce a stroke or cerebral abscess when thrombus or infection bypasses the natural filter of the pulmonary vascular bed. Once an AVM is suspected from radiography, interventional vascular radiology will confirm and delineate the feeding and draining vessels to allow planning for therapeutic embolisation.

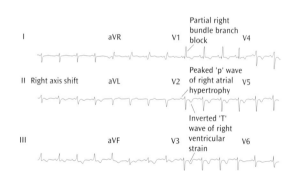

Fig. 1 **ECG of right heart prominence in cor pulmonale.**

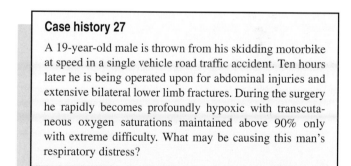

Fig. 2 **Right heart catheterisation with a pulmonory artery flotation catheter and subsequent 'saturation' run.** The catheter is introduced into the superior vena cava, and floated along the blood flow by means of a small air-filled balloon at its distal end. Once through to a pulmonory artery branch, confirmed by pressure tracing characteristics, it is slowly withdrawn. Blood samples are obtained for prompt measurement of oxygen saturation. The example results demonstrate a rise in oxygen saturation in the distal right atrium, in keeping with a left-to-right shunt of oxygenated blood at that site.

Case history 27

A 19-year-old male is thrown from his skidding motorbike at speed in a single vehicle road traffic accident. Ten hours later he is being operated upon for abdominal injuries and extensive bilateral lower limb fractures. During the surgery he rapidly becomes profoundly hypoxic with transcutaneous oxygen saturations maintained above 90% only with extreme difficulty. What may be causing this man's respiratory distress?

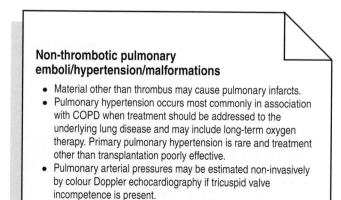

Non-thrombotic pulmonary emboli/hypertension/malformations

- Material other than thrombus may cause pulmonary infarcts.
- Pulmonary hypertension occurs most commonly in association with COPD when treatment should be addressed to the underlying lung disease and may include long-term oxygen therapy. Primary pulmonary hypertension is rare and treatment other than transplantation poorly effective.
- Pulmonary arterial pressures may be estimated non-invasively by colour Doppler echocardiography if tricuspid valve incompetence is present.
- Arteriovenous vascular malformations provide an opportunity for transpulmonary passage of material into the systemic circulation, sometimes with devastating consequences.

PNEUMOTHORAX

The term pneumothorax describes gas, usually air within the pleural space. In most cases air has leaked from alveoli through a defect in the visceral pleura acquired spontaneously or following trauma. Alternatively, air is introduced traumatically from outside. Rarely now is air intentionally introduced into the pleural space to create an artificial pneumothorax, 'resting' the lung in pulmonary tuberculosis before the availability of effective chemotherapy.

The pleural air allows the lung to naturally retract while the chest wall springs out. The consequences for the patient depend on whether the leak continues or the pleural defect seals, and also on the functional state of the underlying lungs. Often the reduction in volume of the recoiling lung is sufficient to bring the edges of the pleural defect into apposition and allow repair. When sealed, the air is slowly re-absorbed across the pleural surface to re-expand the lung.

CLINICAL FEATURES

The main symptoms are sudden-onset pleurisy and undue breathless. The chest pain seems disproportionately severe in young people. Breathlessness is determined by the state of the underlying lung and the size of the pneumothorax. The degree of breathlessness often seems out of proportion to the size of the pneumothorax because of neural reflexes contributing to that sensation. In a patient with severe lung disease and little respiratory reserve, even a small pneumothorax can result in major respiratory distress. The most useful features on examination are reduced chest expansion and reduced breath sounds on the affected side.

CLASSIFICATION AND MECHANISMS

A useful mechanistic classification of pneumothoraces is as follows:

Spontaneous pneumothorax
Primary spontaneous pneumothoraces occur without clear precipitant in a patient without underlying lung disease. The typical patient is a tall thin young male. The underlying defect is a pleural blister-like 'bleb' that is probably congenital. Any pleural weakness would be exacerbated at the lung apices by the more negative intrapleural pressures that are experienced there in tall people. Sometimes these blebs can be seen on a chest radiograph, particularly after the occurrence of a pneumothorax

when the visceral pleura can be seen en face or directly at surgery.

Secondary spontaneous pneumothorax occurs in the presence of underlying acute or chronic lung diseases, occasionally recognised for the first time upon presentation with the pneumothorax. Such pneumothoraces occur by:

- Lung destruction. Staphylococcal infections or tuberculosis can cause direct lung destruction through to the pleura. Infection by *P. carinii* can cause intrapulmonary 'pneumocysts' that can rupture (Fig. 1).
- Gas trapping. All causes of bronchial obstruction especially emphysema or asthma can cause gas trapping and subsequent rupture through bullae. Similar mechanisms apply in fibrotic lung disease, cystic fibrosis and lymphangioleiomyomatosis.

Abnormal connective tissue predisposes in Ehlers–Danlos and in Marfan's syndromes.

Traumatic pneumothorax
Air leaks into the pleura because of a chest wall defect, often a blade wound. Occasionally, chest trauma may cause rib fractures and lung puncture without a skin break. Iatrogenic pneumothoraces occur as a complication of central venous access particularly into the subclavian vein. Other procedures such as intercostal nerve block and transthoracic lung biopsy carry risks of pneumothorax. Pneumothoraces can also be created by mechanical ventilation when large tidal volumes are used to ventilate abnormally stiff lungs, causing 'volutrauma'.

Tension pneumothorax
This term is applied to any pneumothorax that results in cardiopulmonary embarrassment. Usually, it is large pneumothoraces that tension: air continues to leak into the pleural space driven by the thoracic pressure changes of spontaneous or mechanical respiration through a pleural defect functioning as a 'flap valve'. Air moves into the pleural space on inspiration but is prevented from escaping during expiration. The pressure within the pneumothorax then rises displacing the mediastinum, the central vessels deform and cardiac function is impaired. Clinically a poorly moving quiet hemi-thorax with contralateral tracheal deviation are the important signs. At the extreme, electromechanical dissociation and cardiac arrest occur due to obstructed venous return. Occurring in chest trauma victims, haemodynamic deterioration and respiratory distress may be attributed to other injuries. In unconscious patients or those being mechanically ventilated, tension pneumothoraces can be difficult to detect and deserve a high index of suspicion whenever there is cardiorespiratory deterioration.

DIAGNOSIS

Clinical features are non-specific. Except when a patient is deteriorating rapidly, radiology is essential (Fig. 2). On an erect chest radiograph the gas of a pneumothorax should be seen as darker than the adjacent lung and featureless, and bounded by the chest wall and a convex lung edge (Fig. 3). Nevertheless:

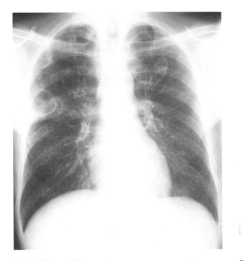

Fig. 1 **X-ray of intrapulmonary pneumocysts.**

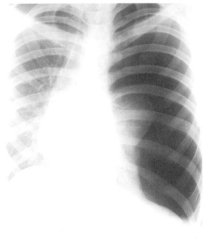

Fig. 2 **Left pneumothorax and pleural blebs visible.**

- A small pneumothorax may be difficult to see. A repeat radiograph taken in full expiration reduces lung volume and makes identification of the unchanged pneumothorax gas volume easier.
- A pneumothorax must be distinguished from a lung bullus. Comparison of previous radiographs is essential and computed tomography useful. Incorrect drainage will result in a bronchopleural fistula which may be difficult to resolve.
- When supine, free pleural gas will collect anteriorly in a cardiophrenic recess. On a chest radiograph even large pneumothoraces may appear subtle. In patients being mechanically ventilated with underlying lung injury such as ARDS, a small pneumothorax may be life threatening. The best imaging modality is CT.

MANAGEMENT

There are two options for the treatment of a pneumothorax: either to allow passive absorption of the intrapleural air and subsequent lung re-expansion or to actively remove the air. The latter can be achieved by transthoracic aspiration through a small bore catheter or by the placement of a wide bore intercostal drainage tube with a one-way valve, usually an underwater seal. In addition it is important to consider any evidence of underlying lung disease. Suspicious symptoms such as haemoptysis or preceeding breathlessness, especially in women, should raise the possibility of rare but important underlying lung diseases.

Radiological review

In small pneumothoraces, radiological observation to complete re-expansion over several weeks is appropriate.

Aspiration

In other cases with near total lung collapse or underlying lung disease, the air should be actively removed by aspiration. This technique is an effective alternative to tube drainage. Should aspiration fail subsequent

Simple pneumothorax	Bulla	Tension pneumothorax	Small pneumothorax
• Dark, featureless • Lung edge visible and convex	• Featureless • Lung edge (pleura) visible and concave • Note angle made with thoracic wall	• Mediastinal shift usual • Clinical haemodynamic compromise	Abnormally stiff lungs may be enough to compromise venous return and hence, cardiac output

Fig. 3 **Radiological distinguishing features of a simple pneumothorax contrasted with a bulla and a tensioning pneumothorax.**

placement of an intercostal tube drain is not precluded.

Intercostal tube drainage

If a tension pneumothorax is suspected, the rapid insertion of an intravenous cannula through the chest wall into the pneumothorax will release the air under pressure, confirm the clinical diagnosis and be life-saving. The definitive drainage tube can then be placed. With traumatic, certainly non-iatrogenic, pneumothoraces an intercostal tube drain should be placed to drain not only air but any blood. These drains are wide bore tubes placed percutaneously under local anaesthetic. Although blunt dissection down to the pleural is standard practice, tubes are available that can be atraumatically placed by means of a Seldinger 'over a wire' technique. Attached to the drainage tube is a one-way valve, usually an underwater seal that remains below the patient's waist. In ambulatory care settings, a Heimlich-style flutter valve is an effective alternative. Such wide bore drains should never be left clamped for fear of the patient developing a covert tension pneumothorax.

Persistent pneumothorax

If the lung remains deflated with a patent chest drain tube then either:

- Air is continuing to leak faster into the pleural space than it can be drained, either via a bronchopleural fistula or from around the tube site itself. The

tube drain will continue to bubble; it should be replaced with the biggest size available.
- The lung itself is prevented from re-expanding by an endobronchial obstruction (mucous plug or tumour) or a thickened cuirass of pleura. In the former case a suction bronchoscopy is required.

The role of continuous low pressure suction is not impressive and can maintain a patent pleural defect by sucking a continuous flow of air from the bronchial tree through the pleural defect and space and out into the drain bottle. Far better is early intervention with surgery or, if not appropriate, the slow healing and re-inflation over several weeks.

Surgery

The place of pleural surgery to obliterate the pleural space and prevent recurrence is established in both recurrent and in contralateral pneumothoraces. It is also indicated at the first pneumothorax if the risk of recurrence is unacceptable, such as for airline pilots. The techniques comprise parietal pleurectomy with pleural abrasion as an adjunct. In addition emphysematous bullae or macroscopically visible pleural defects can be dealt with. In elderly patients, kaolin insufflation under direct vision over the pleura achieves effective pleurodesis. Surgery should only be avoided if lung transplantation could be a future option, such as in cystic fibrosis.

Case history 28

A motorcyclist falls off her bike on the way to catch a transcontinental air flight. Vague chest discomforts ensue but she continues with her journey. An hour into the flight she suffers increasing respiratory distress with worsening chest pain.

What could have happened and why the deterioration?

Pneumothorax

- In rapid onset breathlessness, a pneumothorax should be actively considered.
- A standard good quality chest radiograph is the initial investigation unless there is haemodynamic deterioration when the clinical features of tension should be sought.
- Aspiration is an effective alternative treatment to intercostal tube drainage.
- A pneumothorax may be the presentation of uncommon lung disorders.

PLEURAL EFFUSION

The pleural surfaces of the lung, the chest wall and the mediastinum are lubricated during respiratory movements and cardiac pulsations by pleural surfactant. Lubrication is aided by a thin layer of constantly changing fluid, especially in pleural pockets. Any accumulation of fluid in this potential pleural space is abnormal and represents an effusion.

An accumulation by hydrostatic or oncotic pressure changes will cause fluid relatively poor in protein to collect: a **transudate**. Fluid accumulating by increased inflammatory permeability or obstructed drainage will be protein-rich: an **exudate**.

These two fundamentally different pathophysiological states have clinical importance: a transudate directs diagnostic attention to a systemic problem such as heart failure, whereas an accumulating exudate suggests a local disease process. Unfortunately, this dichotomy is not always perfect.

CLINICAL ASPECTS

History
Pleural effusions are a common respiratory problem, sometimes providing a diagnostic challenge! Progressive breathlessness as the fluid accumulates is the commonest symptom, though pleural pain may be an additional or overshadowing feature. Additional aspects to consider in the history include:

- Smoker – pleural tumour deposits from a lung primary?
- Sudden onset pleurisy – infarction?
- Full occupational history – prior asbestos exposure?
- Systemic disease particularly connective tissue arthritides?
- Abdominal symptoms?

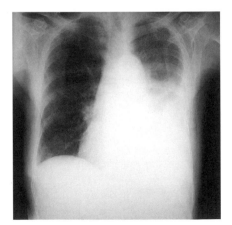

Fig. 1 **Radiograph of pleural effusion.**

Examination
The chest on the effusion side will be poorly expanding and stony dull on percussion, with absent vocal resonance. Remember also that extensive pleural thickening or solid pleural tumour will demonstrate the same physical signs. Look especially for:

- evidence of malignancy elsewhere
- heart failure
- arthritis.

Radiology
Chest radiography may assist in confirming pleural fluid, especially a lateral decubitus view. It rarely identifies the cause unless there are other signs of heart failure such as cardiomegaly or evidence of an underlying pneumonic process. Subpulmonary collections can imitate elevated hemidiaphragms; loculated interlobar fluid may cause confusion appearing as a smooth edged mass that rapidly disappears (pseudotumour). Pleural ultrasound is the most useful investigation to confirm the presence of pleural fluid and site for aspiration. CT scanning can help in complex cases.

CAUSES

The commonest causes in UK clinical practice are indicated in Table 1 and the important distinction between a transudate and an exudate is reaffirmed. This differentiation can often be made on protein levels, blood related to fluid. Similar comparison between lactate dehydrogenase levels often adds little.

CLINICAL INVESTIGATION

The most clinically and diagnostically useful process is to aspirate a sample of the fluid and to obtain biopsies of the parietal pleura. Pleural fluid (30 ml is usually enough) can be aspirated via a 21G needle and dispatched for a range of tests. The appearance of the fluid can provide a clue to its aetiology (Fig. 2):

- Straw-coloured fluid: heart failure, para-pneumonic, malignancy.
- Blood stained: infarction or malignancy.
- Turbid, purulent: empyema.
- Milky: chylous.

The aspirated pleural fluid must undergo further analyses. These include:

- Total protein: < 30g/l indicates transudate; > 30g/l or > 50% total blood protein indicates exudate.
- Lactate dehydrogenase: sometimes helpful in addition to protein concentration for distinguishing transudate from exudate.
- Glucose: low in rheumatoid, para-pneumonic, sometime malignancy.
- Amylase: remains elevated for longer than in blood following pancreatitis.
- Gram's stain: quick and helpful.
- Culture: essential.
- Bacterial antigens pneumococcal CIE useful, is cleared more slowly than from blood in pneumococcal infections.
- Mycobacteria stain and culture though yield is low.
- Differential cell count: useful.
- Malignant cells: essential, though distinguishing reactive from malignant mesothelial cells can be difficult.

Percutaneous pleural biopsies, obtained under local anaesthetic by an Abrams biopsy needle in the presence of

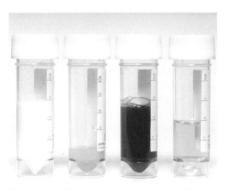

Fig. 2 **Pleural fluid appearances: chyle (milky), pus, blood and straw coloured.**

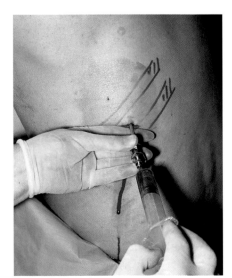

Fig. 3 **Pleural biopsy in progress.**

Table 1 **The most common causes of pleural effusion: transudate vs exudate**

Type	Cause
Transudates	
High venous pressure	Cardiac failure
Low oncotic pressure	Nephrotic syndrome Liver failure* Hypoproteinaemia
Rarities	Hypothyroidism, infarction, peritoneal dialysis*
Exudates	
Malignancy	Lung cancer Secondaries (breast, ovary, GI tract) Mesothelioma Lymphoma
Infarction	Pulmonary embolus
Infection	Para-pneumonic Tuberculosis, primary or post-primary Subphrenic abscess
Inflammatory	Connective tissue (lupus, rheumatoid) Pancreatitis
Obstructive	Chylous
Rarities	Dressler's (post-pericardiotomy post-infarction) syndrome, drugs, sarcoid, benign asbestos pleurisy, Meigs' syndrome,* Yellow-nail syndrome, uraemia

* These abdominal causes reflect the extensive right-side transdiaphragmatic lymphatics present in some individuals that allow pleural fluid to accumulate

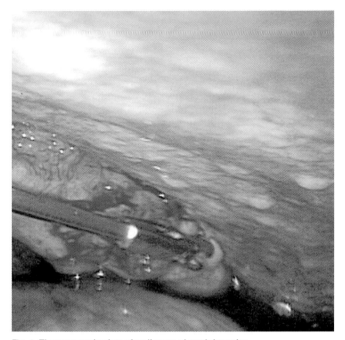

Fig. 4 **Thoracoscopic view of malignant pleural deposits.**
(Copyright Mr. W. S. Walker)

pleural fluid, require a degree of skill in achieving both adequate analgesia and adequate material (Fig. 3). The biopsies should be dispatched both in formalin for histology and fresh (with a drop of sterile saline to prevent drying out) for mycobacterial culture. Percutaneous Abrams biopsies are limited by the blind and random nature of the sampling method. Biopsies of pleura directly visualised at thoracoscopy are more likely to be diagnostic (Fig. 4). This procedure, which can be performed under light sedation and anaesthesia, can also be therapeutic by draining the pleural space and sclerosing once a diagnosis is achieved.

TREATMENT

With transudative effusions, control of the underlying problem will result in reabsortion of the fluid. Very large effusions can be aspirated, taking no more then 1.5 litre at a time to relieve discomfort and breathlessness. More rapid withdrawal can result in a high permeability re-expansion pulmonary oedema.

With exudates, the underlying problem may be treatable. Para-pneumonic effusions should be drained aggressively to dryness. Tuberculosis effusions require standard combination antituberculous chemotherapy with steroids to speed resolution.

With many, particularly malignant, causes, the underlying disease may not be treatable. Relief of breathlessness by drainage and control of fluid re-accumulation is then neces-

sary. Repeated aspirations may suffice. Instilling a non-specific irritant such as kaolin, tetracycline powder (no longer manufactured) or mepacrine may be used to obliterate the pleural space and prevent fluid re-accumulation; a technique known as pleurodesis.

Other important points to consider in treatment include:

- Whenever aspirating pleural fluid, aim to take pleural biopsies at the same time, it may be the only opportunity.

- Apparent 'dry tap' on attempted pleural aspiration:
  —right site?
  —empyema, with viscid material blocking the needle
  —pleural thickening
  —pleural tumour
  —any or all are indications for ultrasound assistance.

- Tips for pleurodesis by tube thoracostomy:
  —can the underlying lung re-expand? If the bronchus is occluded by tumour, pleurodesis will not succeed
  —achieve pleural space dryness both before and 24 hrs after instillation of irritant
  —instil the sclerosant in lignocaine to ease the resulting pleurisy
  —use the procedure early in the disease process; later pleural loculations are more likely.

- Type of primary—breast secondaries seem more amenable to pleural fluid control than lung deposits.

Case history 29

A frail 72-year-old lady presents with breathlessness over 3 weeks. Clinical examination and a chest radiograph confirm a significant right-sided pleural effusion.
What diagnostic procedure should you undertake?
What treatment could you consider if your fears of a malignant cause are confirmed?

Pleural effusion

- Obtain a detailed occupational history in any patient with a unilateral pleural effusion.
- Aspirate **and** biopsy.
- Diagnosis before sclerosis.
- Consider thoracoscopy early.

SLEEP AND SLEEP-DISORDERED RESPIRATION

Sleep-related respiratory disorders have only been appreciated since the early 1980s. There is now increasing interest and understanding of the role that sleep has to play in the mechanisms of chronic, respiratory, ventilatory inadequacy and of primary sleep-related disorders.

STRUCTURE OF SLEEP

Studies of normal subjects sleeping with scalp and facial electrodes to record eye movements (electro-oculography, EOG) and brain activity (electro-encephalograph, EEG) allowed sleep to be divided into rapid eye movement (REM) and non-REM periods of sleep.

REM is sleep characterised by EOG evidence of active eye movements. Muscle tone is greatly diminished in other muscle groups, including respiratory muscles and those involved in maintaining oropharyngeal patency. There is potential for nocturnal underventilation and upper airway closure, especially during REM sleep. In the context of ventilatory failure or upper airway narrowing, sleep will worsen these tendencies.

Non-REM sleep predominates during a normal night's sleep. On the basis of EEG features, it is divided into stages of increasing depth, from drowsiness (stage 0) to deep sleep (stage IV).

UPPER AIRWAY ANATOMY

Above the larynx, a flexible and distensible passage for both respiration and swallowing exists. This need for distensibility challenges patency during inspiration. Nasopharyngeal patency is dependent upon bone and soft tissue dimensions supported by active muscle reflexes.

Below the larynx, the thin-walled, distensible oesophagus runs behind the trachea whose patency is ensured by hoops of cartilage. It is only in the posterior wall of the trachea adjacent to the oesophagus that cartilage is deficient to allow the passage of food boluses.

UPPER AIRWAY COLLAPSE

The gravitational effects of a supine posture together with a narrow nasopharynx may combine to cause upper airway closure during sleep. This is especially likely at the levels of the soft palate and tongue. The basic nasopharyngeal dimensions are genetically determined, including the presence of a posteriorly placed lower jaw (retrognathia). There may be further narrowing by large tonsils or excess soft tissues caused by hypothyroidism, acromegaly or obesity. Alcohol or drugs that sedate or cause muscle relaxation exacerbate the problem (Fig. 1).

OBSTRUCTIVE SLEEP APNOEA (OSA)

OSA is still under-recognised by many medical practitioners and unheard of by the general public. However, it affects at least 1–2% of the female adult population and twice that of men. Obesity is a major factor in the development of the syndrome and with the prevalence of obesity at 50% of the Scottish adult population and expected to increase further, the prevalence of OSA will also increase.

Mechanism and effects

During sleep, especially REM sleep, loss of muscle tone with adverse structural factors leads to pharyngeal collapse. There is a spectrum of effects. At one extreme, narrowing may result in turbulent airflow, tissue vibration and audible snoring but without any daytime consequences, while at the other, complete airway closure results in an obstructive apnoea despite increasing respiratory efforts that usually continue. This apnoea may be prolonged enough to be associated with peripheral blood oxygen desaturation and is terminated by an awakening lasting at most a few seconds but not remembered by the individual. This short awakening, an arousal, recovers upper airway muscular tone and restores patency. Respiratory airflow and sleep then resume. Sometimes resistance to airflow rather than obstruction may be sufficient to cause an arousal and hence sleep disturbance without an apnoea.

This cycle of lost tone, obstructive apnoea and disturbing arousal can occur many times in a night's sleep. With such sleep fragmentation, patients will often complain of unrefreshing nights' sleep, fall asleep readily during the day, and underperform. This tendency to daytime sleeping risks work-related and driving accidents. The associated snoring adds to interpersonal relationship difficulties. The severity of the daytime consequences is not directly related to the degree of nocturnal respiratory disturbance (Fig. 2).

Accompanying each awakening is sympathetic system activation involving tachycardia and an arterial pressure surge. If OSA is untreated for decades, there is now increasing concern of premature vascular disease including coronary and cerebrovascular disease.

Recognition and diagnosis

The key pointers towards the diagnosis are nocturnal snoring, unrefreshing nocturnal sleep and daytime sleeping. Obesity is not a prerequisite, but recent weight gain is common. Indeed, when males gain weight they put more adipose tissue upon their necks, adding to the gravitational load and tendency to upper airway closure.

Confirmation of the diagnosis is required. This currently takes the form of either a home- or hospital-based sleep study to quantify the respiratory abnormalities during sleep (Fig. 3). Suitable equipment may differ in the range of parameters measured and their complexities of detection. However the basis of the diagnosis is to demonstrate:

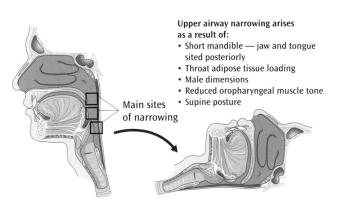

Upper airway narrowing arises as a result of:
• Short mandible — jaw and tongue sited posteriorly
• Throat adipose tissue loading
• Male dimensions
• Reduced oropharyngeal muscle tone
• Supine posture

Main sites of narrowing

Fig. 1 **Factors favouring upper airway collapse during sleep.**

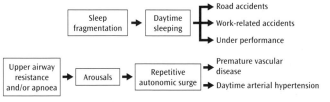

Fig. 2 **Acute and long-term consequences of OSA.**

- upper airway narrowing or closure by sound detection of snoring
  — by thermal or acoustic airflow characteristics
- evidence of arousal as detected
  —by EEG evidence of wakefulness
  — by features of the associated autonomic activation such as heart rate.

Progress is being made in the development of a consistently reliable diagnostic apparatus suitable for home use.

Therapy

Although weight loss and avoidance of evening alcohol or sedating drugs are important, they are rarely sufficient. Identification and correction of endocrine abnormalities should be considered. These manoeuvres will often be insufficient even if attainable.

Splinting the upper airway open during sleep by means of nasally delivered continuous positive airway pressure (CPAP) is usually required. Such therapy delivers an individually titrated pressure with ambient airflow that often requires humidification. The interface between the machine and the individual may be a mask that fits over either the nose or both nose and mouth. Intranasal tubes or cushions are less claustrophobic but often less effective at delivering what amounts to a pneumatic splint. Patient education is an important aspect of therapy. Although the benefits are apparent within a few nights, persevering with such treatment over many years requires motivated and compliant patients and relief of severe daytime symptoms. Readily available technical support is also required.

Surgical techniques to increase the dimensions of the nasopharynx by either trimming the soft palate (uvulopalatopharyngoplasty, U3P) or tensioning the tissues by causing scar tissue

formation (laser palatoplasty) may be tried. However, there are limited, long-term studies demonstrating benefit. Moreover, techniques that trim the palate may make the administration of conventional nasal CPAP more difficult in the future. Dental splinting devices that hold forward either the lower jaw or tongue are more acceptable to many patients reporting mild-to-moderate daytime symptoms and may provide an alternative therapeutic approach.

OTHER CAUSES OF DAYTIME SLEEPING

Any cause of sleep disturbance will result in daytime sleeping. Chiefly affected are night-shift workers, families with newborn babies and patients with nocturnal asthma.

Narcolepsy affects about 0.1% of the population. It is a disorder of REM sleep characterised by irresistible daytime sleeping with, typically, visual hallucinations while falling or awakening from sleep and daytime cataplexy. These patients fall rapidly into REM sleep and there is genetic linkage with HLA-DR2 and -DQ1.

Nocturnal myoclonus – repetitive, sleep-associated, myoclonic limb jerks – causes fragmentation of sleep and, hence, daytime napping. It can be suppressed by benzodiazepine therapy.

Idiopathic hypersomnolence is a diagnosis of exclusion, but may require therapy with stimulant drugs.

NOCTURNAL HYPOVENTILATION

In addition to any tendency for increased upper airway resistance to breathing, the reduction in muscle tone during sleep directly affects the respiratory muscles. Any mechanisms that are operating during wakefulness to compensate for abnormal respiratory mechanics will be disrupted by sleep. The resulting nocturnal hypoventilation is most prominent during REM sleep. Sleep also reduces the

ventilatory drive to hypoxaemia.

In these patients blood CO_2 levels rise during a night's sleep. A headache on awakening owing to the vasodilatation of CO_2 retention is a late sign. Any associated nocturnal hypoxia will stimulate renal erythropoietin secretion and cause a secondary polycythaemia.

Although patients with COPD are the commonest to suffer sleep-related hypoventilation, patients with any cause of respiratory neuromuscular insufficiency are also at risk. Avoidance of drugs and therapies that impair ventilation or upper airway patency is crucial. The addition of chronic, nocturnal, non-invasive, ventilatory support may be required and produces a dramatic improvement in the patients' quality of life and daytime performance.

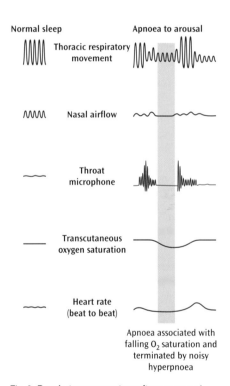

Fig. 3 **Respiratory parameters often measured overnight in the assessment of individuals who might have obstructive sleep apnoea.**

Case history 30

A middle-aged man performing poorly at work and experiencing periods of unresponsiveness, is referred via an occupational physician with concern of 'petit mal' epilepsy. He volunteered that furniture had suffered burn damage at home as a result of napping while smoking. Further questions confirmed long-standing snoring and, with recent weight gain, unrefreshing sleep. His current weight is 121 kg at height 1.68 m and blood pressure 130/85.

What is now required?

Sleep and sleep-disordered respiration

- The most relevant, sleep-associated, respiratory changes are the diminution of muscle tone, especially during REM sleep. This risks both respiratory underventilation and increased upper airway resistance or closure.
- Sleep thus worsens any pre-existing respiratory insufficiency.
- Respiratory abnormalities primarily as a consequence of sleep may cause non-respiratory, daytime symptoms.
- Obstructive sleep apnoea and increased upper airway resistance are under-recognised. Both disturb sleep by repetitive arousals caused by apnoeas or increased respiratory effort. Consider the diagnosis in patients who snore and complain of daytime sleeping and unrefreshing nocturnal sleep.

RESPIRATORY FAILURE

Effective respiration is the moving of environmental oxygen to aerobically metabolising cells and removal of waste carbon dioxide. If this is inadequate, respiratory failure is said to occur.

Respiratory failure has been rather meaninglessly categorised as either type I or type II. More useful is a mechanistic approach to respiratory failure:

- hypoxaemic ($p_aO_2 \leq 8$ kPa) respiratory failure. This threshold relates to the 'knee' of the oxygen–haemoglobin dissociation curve, below which small changes in oxygen partial pressure are associated with large changes in blood oxygen saturation and content.

- hypercapnic ($p_aCO_2 > 6.7$ kPa) ventilatory failure. Although this is often associated with hypoxia, the reverse is not necessarily true. The hypercapnia is not usually immediately life-threatening; much more important is the associated respiratory acidosis.

Such definitions relate to measurements made on arterial blood and reflect the adequacy of tissue delivery or cellular gas exchange.

HYPOXIC RESPIRATORY FAILURE

When airspace flooding occurs with pus, oedema fluid or blood, continued perfusion of non-ventilated lung is functionally equivalent to a shunt. Administration of supplementary inspired oxygen improves the hypoxia with difficulty, as overoxygenation of well-ventilated lung does little to compensate for desaturated blood returning from unventilated lung. Carbon dioxide removal readily occurs via any ventilated area. Chest radiographs are typically white (Fig. 1).

VENTILATORY FAILURE

The respiratory muscle pump can be considered as a neuromuscular pump moving a gas load. Ventilatory failure occurs as a result of either increased load as resistance to movement, or reduced pump capacity or both. The failure may be acute, or an acute deterioration upon chronic insufficiency. A common clinical example is an acute exacerbation of COPD with worsening hypoxaemia and an acute respiratory acidosis. In such patients:

- ventilatory load may be increased – bronchospasm and retained secretions may obstruct ventilation, which adds an additional pressure burden that must be overcome to effect inspiration
- ventilatory capacity may be chronically reduced – muscle wasting and weakness as a result of disuse and poor nutrition often accompanies COPD.

Acute worsening of respiratory muscle function may be by acidosis, sepsis or hypophosphataemia and impaired neural respiratory drive by hypercapnic somnolence, sedating drugs or sleep (Fig. 2).

Management includes oxygenation and support to allow the underlying causes to be identified and treated specifically. Hypoxaemia here is readily corrected by supplementary oxygen. The associated hypercapnia and ventilatory inadequacy require addressing and patients may require additional ventilatory support. The common reluctance to adequately oxygenate many patients with chronic lung disease, especially COPD, for fear of removing their 'hypoxic' drive to ventilation is inappropriate. In reality, very few patients are dependent on such a drive. Chest radiographs are typically dark.

RESPIRATORY FAILURE WITH SEPSIS

Typically there is impaired, intracellular utilisation of oxygen and vascular maldistribution such that need may outstrip supply locally. Products from the infecting organism and the host's response are responsible.

CLINICAL MANAGEMENT

Hypoxaemia and ventilatory failure are the two commonest causes of respiratory failure. Their clinical management can usefully be considered as the two issues of correcting hypoxia and supporting ventilation with the setting of both therapeutic goals and appropriate monitoring of each.

Oxygen therapy

In healthcare environments pressurised oxygen is often available piped from tanks. Cylinders are also available but they do not last long and pose difficulties in delivery and manoeuvrability. Liquid oxy-

gen in robust, insulated flasks or oxygen concentrators that extract oxygen from environmental air are more usual alternatives for home use.

There are a number of patient interfaces.

Low flow rates, up to 4 lpm for short periods, can be delivered by **nasal cannulae**. These are more comfortable and less claustrophobic than masks, and are more likely to provide continuous oxygen enrichment during eating, talking or drinking. They are the most useful for home use and when low levels of enrichment are needed during exacerbations of COPD. However, the inspired oxygen fraction is indeterminate and varies with the patient's own minute ventilation that is itself variable. There is thus a need for careful titration and monitoring with pulse oximetry and blood gas estimations in the unstable acutely ill patient and upon initiating chronic therapy in the stable patient.

Oxygen masks have the superficial attraction of being tailored to deliver a predetermined oxygen concentration dependent on the oxygen flow rate and a venturi valve. However the higher the level of oxygen enrichment required, the

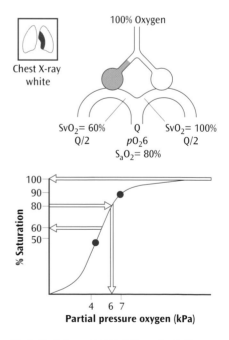

Fig. 1 **Hypoxic respiratory failure: shunt.** Diagram illustrates the disproportionate effect on efferent blood pO_2 that the shunted flow has, due to the shape of the oxygen–haemoglobin dissociation curve.
Q = cardiac output, 1/2 to the ventilated portion.
Extensive consolidation and inflammation counteracts hypoxic vasoconstriction as regards blood flow distribution.

more unlikely it is to be achieved unless the mask volume is large or a reservoir bag is used. Even at flow rates of 10–15 lpm, ill patients with high minute ventilation are likely to have inspiratory flow rates easily in excess of that deliverable.

Careful assessment of this therapy is required. Transcutaneous pulse oximetry probes are now robust and are a useful real-time assessment of peripheral arterial blood oxygen saturation if peripheral circulation is adequate. Measurement of the adequacy of ventilation is still necessary by arterial puncture and p_aCO_2 measurement, as current transcutaneous sensors are poor responders to change, uncomfortable and not readily available. It is important to remember that adequate oxygenation can be achieved in the face of life-threateningly inadequate ventilation.

Compressed oxygen is anhydrous and high flow rates for even short periods are very drying to the respiratory tract and require active humidification. Lower flows used for chronic treatment can be just as drying too. As in any therapeutic intervention, the goal of oxygen therapy is clearly to relieve hypoxaemia without using unnecessary high or prolonged exposure to oxygen that is toxic. The actual target will vary between patients: those with chronic hypoxia will require supplementation to a lower level of oxygenation, ideally individualised but at least to the 'knee' of the oxygen dissociation curve.

Ventilatory support

Respiratory stimulants. The only respiratory stimulant in routine clinical use is doxapram, which is usually administered by continuous infusion. It has a place in the management of acute-on-chronic respiratory failure in exacerbations of COPD. It stimulates both peripheral and central chemosensitive receptors to increase minute ventilation. If ventilatory failure is the result of an opiate excess or pure benzodiazepine overdose, then use of the specific antagonists naloxone and flumazenil will reverse the ventilatory inadequacy. However, both are short-acting drugs that may require repeated administration.

Non-invasive mechanical ventilation (nIPPV). This has been a welcome development in respiratory critical care over the last decade. Such devices administer positive pressure support, via a nasal or full-face mask, to augment a patient's ventilatory activity. Such ventilation avoids the risks of tracheal intubation and aids weaning, but patients may be intolerant of the mask and airway protection is inadequate if vomiting occurs. It may also avoid the utilisation of intensive care resources and is an alternative or additional option to doxapram infusion in managing acute-on-chronic ventilatory failure. Much of the technology and expertise has developed from nasal CPAP therapy for obstructive sleep apnoea. The experience with nIPPV has continued to grow, especially for acidotic exacerbations of COPD or neuromuscular conditions leading to ventilatory insufficiency with chronic domiciliary support.

Mechanical ventilatory support. Mechanical ventilation developed as negative pressure 'iron lungs' to provide long-term respiratory support for survivors of poliomyelitis and paralysing encephalitis infections. These ventilators enclosed much of the torso and by cycling a vacuum would draw air into the lungs. Passive recoil following loss of the vacuum allowed expiration. The equipment required tends to be large.

The development of tracheal intubation, by means of oral, nasal and percutaneous routes, allowed cycling positive pressure for ventilation during anaesthesia for surgery. Development of both ventilation and sedation techniques has allowed respiratory support for critically ill patients to be provided outwith operating theatre anaesthesia. Positive pressure ventilation is now the usual support provided. It requires tracheal intubation or tracheostomy and connection to a mechanical ventilator. The ventilation parameters are adjustable and as current machines allow patients to attempt their own respiration, heavy sedation or paralysis of patients is not now routinely required. Short-term ventilation of up to a couple of weeks is achieved with minimally traumatic cuffed endotracheal tubes. Longer-term ventilation is more comfortably provided by placement of a tube via a tracheostomy. Provision of the required technical equipment with appropriate medical and nursing support is usually only possible in dedicated intensive care units.

Factors to consider:
- **Respiratory drive**
  - sedative or analgesic drugs
  - sleep
- **Neuromuscular load**
  - neuromuscular disease or atrophy
  - electrolyte disturbance
  - drugs impairing function
- **Airway resistance**
  - secretion
  - bronchospasm
  - upper airway collapse

Chest X-ray dark

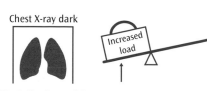

Fig. 2 **Ventilatory failure.**

Case history 31

A 57-year-old man is mechanically ventilated for his first-ever hospital admission with an infective exacerbation of COPD. His only other medical problem is long-standing alcohol dependence. On weaning he struggles to adequately self-ventilate. Serum potassium remains at 3.2 mM despite copious parenteral supplements and serum phosphate is noted to be less than 0.5 mM.

Comments?

Respiratory failure

- Measure arterial blood gases in ill patients. Address oxygenation and ventilation as separate but related issues, each with its own therapy and goals. Inadequate correction of hypoxia for fear of worsening ventilatory drive is incorrect and inappropriate.
- Adequately relieved hypoxaemia may co-exist with life-threatening ventilatory inadequacy and respiratory acidosis.
- The causes of acute ventilatory failure, especially exacerbations of COPD, are often multifactorial. All need considering and attempts made at correction. Temporary respiratory support with doxapram and/or non-invasive ventilation may be required.
- Treat oxygen as any other drug: determine aim(s) of treatment, prescribe appropriately and monitor effectiveness.

SURGICAL TECHNIQUES/TRANSPLANTATION

THORACIC SURGERY

Thoracic surgeons are crucial members of any respiratory team. The last couple of decades has seen lung transplantation mature as a treatment option, thoracoscopic developments at the leading edge of 'key hole' surgery and novel lung reduction techniques devised for patients with severe pulmonary emphysema.

Thoracoscopy

Traditionally, a single, rigid, viewing scope with an operating channel is inserted percutaneously into the pleural space. The presence of pleural fluid or air eases access but previous pleurisy may make it impossible. Thoracoscopy allows both pleural surfaces to be inspected, biopsies to be taken and insufflation of a sclerosant for pleurodesis.

With the advent of video-image assistance, more complicated surgical techniques, including pneumonectomy, can now be performed (Fig. 1). Three 'ports' are placed percutaneously, usually in the lateral chest: one for viewing and two for instrumentation. Such minimally invasive surgery might require longer operating and anaesthetic times but often the patient has a quicker post-operative recovery. Use of this technique for lung biopsy has encouraged the earlier and more frequent acquisition of histological material in patients with interstitial lung disease.

Mediastinal assessment

The adequate staging of patients with potentially resectable lung cancer may require preliminary surgical assessment of the mediastinum. Similar surgical techniques are utilised to obtain pathological material from the mediastinum when malignancy is but one possibility.

In mediastinoscopy, a narrow, rigid, tubular mediastinoscope is inserted in the suprasternal notch. Careful, blunt, pretracheal dissection with small swabs at a distance allows the instrument to advance for paratracheal node sampling, often as far as the subcarinal area.

Mediastinotomy is an incision through a left interspace, allowing access to the left mediastinum and hilum under the aortic arch. This technique is more usually performed for directed biopsy rather than mediastinal assessment.

Lung resection

Lobe or lung resection with removal of draining hilar nodes in patients with lung cancer is limited to those in whom prior staging has demonstrated that such surgical resection will be complete. Careful, clinical, laboratory and radiological staging is required to demonstrate absence of disease spread. Formal mediastinal assessment is often required too. In addition, patients must be fit enough for such major surgery with its requirement for single lung ventilation during the anaesthetic. They must have sufficient respiratory

reserve for the planned lung resection and be free of underlying diseases with important anaesthetic implications. 'Open and close' thoracotomies for malignancy should be rare on any unit.

Surgery for benign disease is not common. Indications include resection of localised bronchiectasis or other areas of chronic suppuration. Solitary lesions removed because of a concern of malignancy may turn out to be benign, often tuberculous or fungal.

Peri- and post-operative complications are more likely in patients who smoke immediately pre-operatively and in those with poor underlying pulmonary function or important co-morbidities, especially ischaemic heart disease. Specific post-operative complications include:

- Sputum retention with lobar collapse.
- Acute respiratory distress syndrome in the contralateral lung. This may be the result of an entire cardiac output with pro-inflammatory mediators passing through its vascular bed during the single lung anaesthesia and surgery.
- Bronchial stump blow-out following pneumonectomy allows air and infection into the pneumonectomy space. It is suggested by the arrest of the normal progression of an air–fluid level up the pneumonectomy space on serial chest radiographs. It can be life-threatening if the stump defect

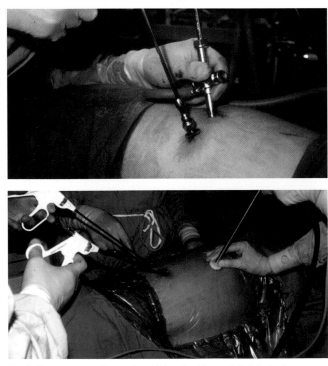

Fig. 1 **Thoracoscopy. Conventional (above); video-assisted (below).** (Copyright Mr. W. S. Walker.)

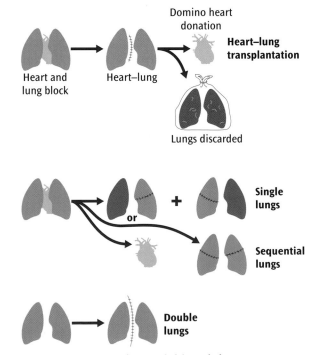

Fig. 2 **Heart and lung transplantations maximising gain from a scarce resource.**

allows the pneumonectomy space contents to spill back into the normal lung. Infection can never be eradicated from the pneumonectomy space and a lifetime of empyema and tube drainage results. When this develops after resection for tumour, the patient's survival may be enhanced. Surgical techniques to reduce its likelihood include filling the stump with biocompatible glue in addition to double rows of staples or sutures.

- Post-thoracotomy pain is a persistent, neuralgic pain, sometimes incapacitating, which may occur as a result of intra-operative irritation or bruising of the intercostal nerve at thoracotomy or thoracoscopy. Its occurrence may be reduced by pre-emptive analgesia.

Transplantation

This is now an acceptable form of treatment for suitable patients with chronic progressive lung and pulmonary vascular diseases, especially interstitial pulmonary fibrosis, cystic fibrosis and emphysema. A single lung or a heart–lung block can be transplanted. Bilateral sepsis in cystic fibrosis requires sequential single lung transplantation. There may be the opportunity to transplant the recipient's heart onward in a domino fashion. Severe right heart disease is likely to require a heart–lung donor block (Fig. 2).

Despite vigorous patient selection, the peri-operative mortality is high but overall 50–60% survive to 5 years. The long-term problems of chronic rejection and of infection from the legacy of lifelong immunosuppression remain current concerns following any organ transplant.

As with any transplant programme, the availability of donor organs remains the major limitation to this form of therapy. The surgical techniques themselves are designed to maximise organs available for transplantation. Consideration of lobe donation from a living donor has been

explored in paediatric practice. The ethics and practicalities of developing genetically human lungs in donor animals remain to be solved.

Surgery for pulmonary emphysema

Transplantation remains at least a theoretical, if not a practical, surgical option.

Bullectomy. Removal of a bulla by deflation and ligation or stapling as bullectomy is usually only of benefit if it is causing compression of adjacent lung tissue. This requires pre-operative assessment by CT scanning and occasionally by isotope ventilation and perfusion lung scanning. Bullae usually occur in the presence of diffuse bullous lung disease and removal of the largest bulla does not always compensate for the respiratory abnormalities of the remaining lung tissue.

Lung volume reduction (Fig. 3). Tissue is trimmed bilaterally from hyperinflated lungs. This reduction in lung volume allows the diaphragm to revert towards a more normal domed appearance and the respiratory muscles to operate at a better mechanical advantage. That the surgery works is demonstrated by improvement both subjectively and objectively in terms of gas transfer and walking distances. However, its place in the long-term management of patients with COPD, particularly in relation to formal exercise rehabilitation programmes, is as yet unclear.

Bronchoscopy

Rigid bronchoscopy is a technique usually performed by thoracic surgeons under general anaesthesia. It has the attractions of ensuring adequate oxygenation and control of the airway with good images albeit of only the very central airways. It is the best technique to control bleeding as suction obtained through the wide channel of a rigid scope is substantial. In addition, biopsies are big, foreign body retrieval is usually easy and assessment of the mobility of the airways is possible.

By contrast, **flexible bronchoscopy** is more widely available and is often performed by thoracic physicians under local anaesthesia with intravenous sedation. Routine use of pulse oximetry and supplementary oxygen minimises the risks of hypoxia. It is mainly a diagnostic tool, allowing inspection of the major airways and obtaining biopsies of central endobronchial lesions or more distal parenchymal lung biopsies.

There is now increasing interest in the therapeutic techniques able to be performed via flexible rather than rigid bronchoscopes. These include the placement of stents and radio-active sources, resection of endobronchial tissue by laser or cautery and retrieval of inhaled objects by snares. Many of these techniques can be used to palliate some of the most distressing symptoms of lung cancer, especially breathlessness. The range of therapeutic possibilities has been increased by the miniaturisation of endoscopic equipment. There is a relative maximal size of these scopes, determined in part by the airway dimensions and the requirement for adequate ventilation around them. Within this maximum, light source, image lens or videochip and operating/suction channel all have to fit.

Case history 32

A middle-aged man with severe bullous emphysema, gas transfer (T_{Lco}) barely 25% of predicted and a 6-minute walking distance of 103 m is referred to a regional cardiothoracic unit for consideration of lung transplantation. After a period of inpatient assessment, he accepts the suggestion of staged bilateral lung volume reduction surgery. Surgery is completed successfully. Upon review 6 months later, he reports subjective benefit, T_{Lco} remains 24% of predicted but he now walks 190 m in 6 minutes.

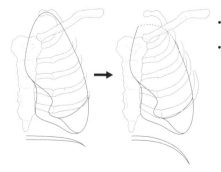

Fig. 3 **Lung volume reduction surgery.**

- Upper lobes 'trimmed' surgically
- Ribs and diaphragm working at a better mechanical advantage

Surgical techniques/transplantation

- Thoracic surgeons are crucial team members, and only they can truly determine the operability of patients with lung cancer.
- Much of their work is cancer surgery, but there have been exciting developments in video-assistance, thoracoscopic surgery, lung volume reduction and transplantation.
- Techniques are developing for palliation of lung cancer symptoms via rigid and, increasingly, flexible bronchoscopes.

THE LUNG IN ADVERSE ENVIRONMENTS

HIGH ALTITUDE

Hypoxia and cold are the main challenges of high altitude. With increasing altitude, the partial pressure of oxygen falls exponentially with atmospheric pressure, halving every 5500 m (Fig. 1). Before Messner and Habeler reached the summit of Mount Everest (8848 m) in 1978 without supplementary oxygen it had been considered impossible. Even their brief spell on the summit was characterised by the neuropsychiatric sequelae of extreme hypoxia. Extremes of altitude are reached only by a few mountaineers and indigenous herdsmen, but increasing numbers of travellers and winter sportsmen ascend, often rapidly, to levels of altitude that risk medical complications. There are few physiological studies on the indigenous people of high altitude. The results of studies on lowlanders moving to altitude are likely to reflect the complex interactions between rates of ascent, altitude, exercise and dehydration.

With acute exposure to altitude, there is a rapid and maintained increase in minute ventilation. The ensuing respiratory alkalosis is accompanied by compensatory renal bicarbonate loss. The hypoxia causes generalised pulmonary vasoconstriction, which improves ventilation–perfusion matching, but only during rest. These changes are paralleled by an increased cardiac output and peripheral vasoconstriction shifting oxygen delivery towards the central circulation.

Longer term residence results in increasing haematocrit, which is a result of

nocturnal hypoventilation and worsening hypoxia that stimulates erythropoietin secretion. Exercise in the relatively dry atmosphere at altitude will cause dehydration and intravascular volume contraction. There is an increase in muscle capillaries, myoglobin and mitochondria that may be partially explained by the muscle wasting that occurs at altitude. Residents of the high plateau are polycythaemic, and suffer from chronic pulmonary hypertension.

High altitude syndromes

The high altitude syndromes reflect inadequate physiological adaptation, acclimatisation, as a result of too rapid an ascent. There are wide inter-individual variations in safe rates of ascent. The only rules are to 'climb high, sleep low', and to descend if unwell. There are several common high altitude syndromes:

- Acute mountain sickness (AMS) is common and occurs within a few hours of rapid ascent to above 2500 m. It is predominantly neurological, with lassitude, fluid retention, anorexia and a vasogenic headache the main symptoms. There is measurable pulmonary dysfunction as a result of interstitial fluid. At least a quarter of individuals going to this altitude will complain of these effects. Slower ascent and acetazolamide (mild diuretic and respiratory stimulant properties) help.
- High altitude pulmonary oedema (HAPE) may follow AMS or occur de novo. It is a non-cardiogenic high permeability oedema resulting from disruption of the alveolar–capillary membrane. This is a result of the shear stresses induced when increased cardiac output is delivered into the

vasoconstricted hypoxic pulmonary vascular bed. There is also an inflammatory response which adds to the damage. It can be fatal and requires prompt recognition and rapid descent with oxygen therapy. Temporary relief may be obtained with a portable hyperbaric chamber, if available (Fig. 2). Prevention by ascending slowly is preferable.

- High altitude cerebral oedema occasionally occurs in conjunction with HAPE. Untreated, it is rapidly fatal. Management and prevention are the same as for HAPE.

AIR PASSENGER TRANSPORT

Increasingly, patients with chronic respiratory disabilities wish to fly. Assistance on the ground through large, and often crowded, airport terminals is often required for embarkation and disembarkation of patients with impaired exercise tolerance. Once airborne, medical incidences on commercial flights are rare, at about 2 out of 100 000 passengers, one-half being cardiac in nature. As respiratory events are less dramatic, the 10% reported may well be an underestimate. The specific respiratory risks of commercial passenger flights are:

- **Hypoxia.** Aircraft cabins are pressurised to a compromise between ground level and cruising altitude, usually to the equivalent of 1000–2400 m. This lowers the ambient partial pressure of oxygen to 15–17 kPa, thereby reducing alveolar oxygen tensions with resulting hypoxaemia. It is difficult to predict the arterial oxygenation of patients with lung disease at such altitude but attempts have been made to predict p_aO_2 at rest for patients with stable COPD and restrictive lung disease using equations generated by volunteer patients breathing hypoxic gas mixtures. In general, patients who are hypercapnic or substantially hypoxaemic (p_aO_2 below ~6.6 kPa) at sea level should not fly without support. With advanced warning, many of the major carrier airlines can arrange for supplementary oxygen to be available in-flight, separate from the cabin's emergency supply.
- **Cabin air quality.** Cabin air is a recirculating mixture of 'used' interior air mixed with warmed, but extremely dry, external air, usually extracted from the engine intakes. The low humidity

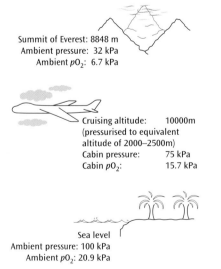

Summit of Everest: 8848 m
Ambient pressure: 32 kPa
Ambient pO_2: 6.7 kPa

Cruising altitude: 10000m
(pressurised to equivalent altitude of 2000–2500m)
Cabin pressure: 75 kPa
Cabin pO_2:   15.7 kPa

Sea level
Ambient pressure: 100 kPa
Ambient pO_2: 20.9 kPa

Fig. 1 **Effect of altitude.** Ambient pressure drops roughly linearly from sea level (100 kPa) to 110 000 m and oxygen percentage remains static. Hence, the ambient partial pressure of oxygen remains 20.9% of the ambient pressure.

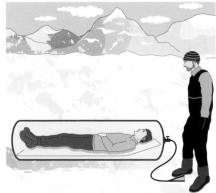

Fig. 2 **Portable altitude chamber.** This portable hyperbaric chamber is able to pressurise an individual to a few atmospheres by foot pump.

risks dehydrating passengers, especially on long haul flights, and is a risk compounded by alcoholic beverages. The quality of cabin air is detrimentally affected by the degree of re-use; hence the risks of passive smoke inhalation and respiratory infections. There is a real risk of airborne infections, especially viral, including documented transmission of drug-resistant tuberculosis.

- **Pulmonary thrombiemboli.** Travellers are at increased risk of developing deep venous thrombosis as a consequence of immobility with vascular stasis and of relative dehydration. This is an especial risk on long flights in the more cramped accommodation of economy class. The use of pre-flight prophylactic aspirin has been suggested.

- **Pneumothoraces.** Pneumothoraces developing in-flight are rare. Pneumothoraces developing on the ground before flying are a medical contraindication to flight, as is recent pleural surgery. The lower cabin pressure will allow the pleural gas volume to expand with a real risk of cardiovascular compromise and death. Media interest in in-flight saviours should not overshadow the fact that the passenger should never have flown in the first place.

SPACE TRAVEL

Astronauts and space station personnel are cocooned in a pressurised, oxygenated and warm local environment. The minimal gravity present has beneficial respiratory effects. The work of breathing may be reduced. Moreover, the gravitationally induced pulmonary blood flow gradient is absent. Hence pulmonary perfusion is even better matched to ventilation. However, 'weightlessness' rapidly results in loss of cardiovascular vasoconstricting reflexes. Upon return to earth, the resulting profound postural hypotension is incapacitating.

DEPTH, DIVING AND DECOMPRESSION

With increasing depth under water, gas volume is compressed. Each 10 m of depth is equal to one atmosphere in pressure. Trained skindivers overcoming buoyancy can descend to around 25 m in a single breath-hold dive. The stimulus to rebreathing is more thoracic sensory stimuli than rising carbon dioxide. Sports, and many professional, divers breathe compressed air underwater, delivered to them via a demand valve at ambient pressure (Fig. 3). With increasing depth, the increasing pressures dissolve substantial amounts of nitrogen into body fat and, particularly, neural tissue. It behaves as an anaesthetic, resulting in disinhibition ('rapture of the deep'), drowsiness and coma ('inert gas narcosis'). This limits pleasure diving breathing air to around 30 m. Replacing the nitrogen by oxygen is not an alternative as pulmonary and neural toxicity occurs. Helium is a suitable substitute.

Having dived to depth, most medical problems arise during ascent and re-surfacing. Falling ambient pressure allows intrathoracic gas volume to expand, developing shear stresses and risking intrapulmonary rupture. The lowering partial pressure of nitrogen may allow it to come out of solution and form gas bubbles, particularly in the capillary and venous circulations. Either mechanism may result in intravascular gas bubbles and their embolisation. These bubbles may coalesce and will expand with further falls in pressure. The manifestations of intravascular gas are termed 'decompression illness'. The bubbles cause vascular obstruction with tissue necrosis and symptoms including pain. There is a predilection for articular ('the bends'), pulmonary (infarction-like), or neurological sites.

Pulmonary barotrauma consequent on expanding gas volumes rupturing peri-bronchially or pleura may also present as pneumothoraces or pneumo-mediastinum. This is more likely in abnormal lungs when airways obstruction will delay pressure equalisation, or localised fibrosis, being less pliant, will rupture.

Prevention is better than cure. Divers need to adequately vent their lungs upon ascending, and the rate of ascent must be sufficiently slow to allow inert gases to leach out from tissues without forming bubbles. After deep professional dives, staged 'decompression' periods are required at depth; safe ascents may require days. Decompression complications require treatment of re-pressurisation with oxygen therapy upon surfacing. Pressure tanks are rare in most countries and rapid transportation to hyperbaric chambers is required. Even after an uneventful dive and ascent, immediate air travel should be avoided since the risks of ascent continue when the aeroplane decompresses climbing to altitude.

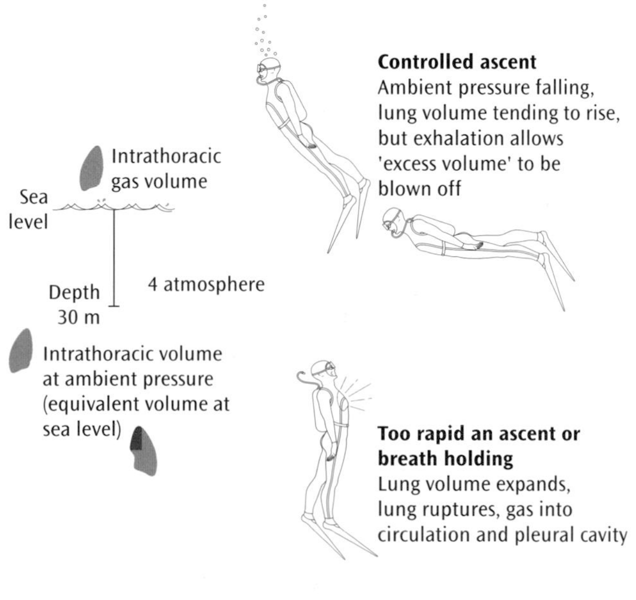

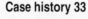

Sea level

Intrathoracic gas volume

Depth 30 m   4 atmosphere

Intrathoracic volume at ambient pressure (equivalent volume at sea level)

Controlled ascent
Ambient pressure falling, lung volume tending to rise, but exhalation allows 'excess volume' to be blown off

Too rapid an ascent or breath holding
Lung volume expands, lung ruptures, gas into circulation and pleural cavity

Fig. 3 **Lung volumes and depth.**

Case history 33

A teenager returns from his first holiday abroad by plane. As the aircraft climbs after takeoff he becomes increasingly breathless, light headed and is noted by his companions to be blue. He remains distressed until the aircraft descends to land at Edinburgh airport, when he is brought to hospital. What would you expect to find?

The lung in adverse environments

- Acclimatisation to altitude involves progressive increase in ventilation over days and progressive polycythaemia over weeks. Too rapid an ascent to altitude risks life-threatening pulmonary and cerebral oedema.
- The presence of a pneumothorax, recent subaqua diving or severe respiratory failure are contraindications to commercial aircraft flight.

RADIOLOGICAL TECHNIQUES AND SUPPORT

Clinical respiratory medicine is crucially dependent on the support which radiology offers in a range of imaging and interventional techniques.

PLAIN CHEST RADIOGRAPHY

The centred and correctly exposed erect postero-anterior (PA) chest radiograph can be considered part of the respiratory clinical examination. It requires skill in both obtaining and interpretation. Films taken by portable equipment are often antero-posterior or supine in orientation and may be of a lesser quality. Their correct interpretation often requires even greater skill.

Recent developments in radiology have affected even the plain chest films. A technique of fragmenting X-ray beams and subsequent equalisation of exposures (AMBER) increases the detail visible through the heart and below the diaphragms. Digital image processing allows radiology departments to miniaturise, store and rapidly retrieve chest radiograph images.

Notwithstanding these newer techniques, inspection of any previous chest radiographs is essential in the investigation of any patient with an abnormal radiograph. Films are rarely kept indefinitely because of space and weight. There is also retrievable silver in the film emulsions, but storage for 5–10 years is usual.

TOMOGRAPHY

By moving both the X-ray emitting tube and radiation sensor through circular arcs, an image is produced which is focused on the centre of rotation; structures above and below are blurred out (Fig. 1). Conventional tomography has largely been superseded by computed techniques. However, conventional techniques are more widely available and can produce diagnostically useful information about intrapulmonary masses and cavities (p. 30).

Computed tomography (CT) requires both tube and detector to revolve completely around the patient. Radiodensity information is obtained on each revolution and subsequent analysis generates detailed image 'slices' orientated transversely and displayed as an image with picture elements displaying average radiodensities on a grey scale.

Usual CT scans of the thorax produce images based on information obtained from contiguous 10 mm slices every 10 mm. Intravascular injection of contrast will opacify vascular structures. Once acquired the images can be manipulated to demonstrate either the lungs or the more radiodense (beam attenuating) tissues of thoracic cage and mediastinum (p. 38).

High resolution CT scanning uses the same principles but acquires radiodensity information to produce tissue images of one or two millimetres every 15 mm. Not all the thorax is imaged yet diagnostic and therapeutically useful information is obtained on diffuse pulmonary conditions including emphysema and interstitial lung diseases. This technique is more sensitive than a chest radiograph in detecting early diffuse parenchymal disease (p. 42), though small solitary lesions may easily be missed.

Spiral CT scanning visualises the whole thorax volume. The scanning equipment moves continuously around the gantry feeding the patient into the scanner rather than stopping between each image acquisition. Thus the scanned volume is sampled entirely in a helical fashion. Compared to conventional CT scanning, imaging is much quicker and radiation dose may be less. Moreover as the whole tissue volume is scanned, image reconstruction in any plane or in three dimensions is possible. In conjunction with intravascular contrast, the image quality may allow thrombus within central pulmonary arteries to be visualised (Fig. 2).

MAGNETIC RESONANCE (MR) IMAGING

Powerful electromagnetic pulses cause temporary shifts in proton orientation within the nuclei of tissues being studied. These shifts and their subsequent recovery emit radio signals which are utilised to produce images. Lung and many mediastinal MR images lack the detail that CT can provide. However, in selected cases, the technique can provide very useful information about the mediastinum, spine and chest wall (Fig. 3).

ULTRASOUND

Ultrasound does not penetrate aerated lung. However, it is non-ionising radiation and the acoustic reflections allow useful imaging of the pleura, adjacent structures and the heart. Here spatial resolution is better than CT imaging. Confirming the presence of pleural fluid or a solid pleural abnormality is especially useful in cases of a 'dry' pleural tap. A transthoracic cardiac ultrasound examination can provide quantitative and qualitative information on ventricular and valve performance. Such an assessment is useful in the investigation of otherwise unexplained breathlessness. If

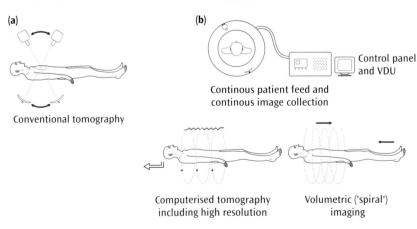

(a)

Conventional tomography

(b)

Control panel and VDU

Continous patient feed and continous image collection

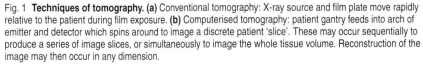

Computerised tomography including high resolution

Volumetric ('spiral') imaging

Fig. 1 **Techniques of tomography. (a)** Conventional tomography: X-ray source and film plate move rapidly relative to the patient during film exposure. **(b)** Computerised tomography: patient gantry feeds into arch of emitter and detector which spins around to image a discrete patient 'slice'. These may occur sequentially to produce a series of image slices, or simultaneously to image the whole tissue volume. Reconstruction of the image may then occur in any dimension.

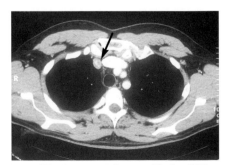

Fig. 2 **CT pulmonary angiogram with clot visible in right pulmonary artery (arrowed).**

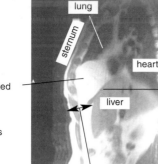

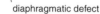

Fig. 3 **MRI of diaphragmatic hernia.**

tricuspid valve incompetence is present, an estimate of pulmonary arterial pressures can be made. Transoesophageal ultrasound techniques are especially useful in generating images of the left atrium and adjacent mediastinal structures.

ISOTOPE IMAGING

Isotope imaging utilises gamma emitting medical isotopes with short radioactive half lives as tracers. Following intravenous injection or inhalation, their distribution and accumulation can be followed by gamma camera imaging that lacks detailed spatial resolution.

Lung ventilation can be semi-quantitatively studied by either attaching a tracer such as technetium–99m (^{99m}Tc) to nebulisable particles or utilising a short half-life radioactive gaseous isotope such as xenon. Measuring regional ventilation can help in the assessment of lung function and estimation of residual function following lung or lobe resection for tumour or resecting emphysematous bullae.

Intravenously re-injecting albumin attached to an appropriate tracer will be delivered to the pulmonary vascular bed and can thereby image lung perfusion. The presence of perfusion defects may suggest vessel occlusion as in pulmonary thromboemboli or vascular bed closure due to hypoxic vasoconstriction consequent on other lung disease. This may be a developing pneumonia, causing a local abnormality, or airways obstruction. Hence, a plain chest radiograph and knowledge of the patient's pulmonary function is crucial in the correct interpretation of isolated perfusion scans in particular. More usual is combined perfusion with ventilation scans for the diagnosis of pulmonary emboli by demonstrating perfusion defects mismatched to any ventilation defects.

Phosphate isotopes taken up by bone are used in bone scintigraphy imaging. Localised accumulation occurs in both benign and malignant bone diseases, but correlated with plain radiographic appearances the technique is useful in the evaluation of bone pain in patients with malignant disease (Fig. 4).

ANGIOGRAPHY

Pulmonary arteries can be accessed from the femoral vein via the right heart. The selective catheterisation of pulmonary vessels followed by intravascular contrast injection is considered the gold standard in the investigation of pulmonary emboli. The risks to the patient with modern flexible catheters and current radiocontrast media are very slight.

INTERVENTIONAL RADIOLOGY

This is a developing area of pulmonary radiology. Here are a few examples:

- intravascular embolisation with metal coils of bleeding bronchial arteries to stem life-threatening haemoptysis
- ultrasound guided placement of drainage catheters into pleural empyemas
- percutaneous CT guided lung biopsy of peripheral lesions requiring a tissue diagnosis but where surgical resection is not possible (p. 55)
- intravascular stenting of the superior vena cava which rapidly relieves the symptoms of obstruction
- placement of stents (Fig. 5).

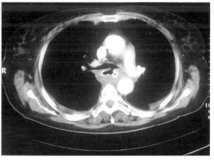

(a)

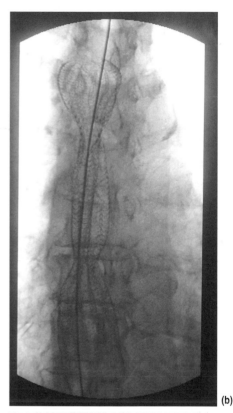

(b)

Fig. 5 **Interventional stent. (a)** CT at level of a (malignant) fistula between oesophagus and left main stem bronchus. **(b)** Metal stents with radiolucent covering attempting to seal the fistula into the left main stem bronchus.

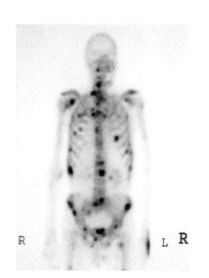

Fig. 4 **Isotope bone scan.**

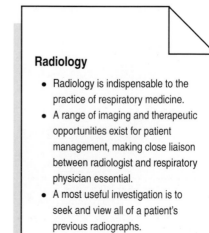

Radiology

- Radiology is indispensable to the practice of respiratory medicine.
- A range of imaging and therapeutic opportunities exist for patient management, making close liaison between radiologist and respiratory physician essential.
- A most useful investigation is to seek and view all of a patient's previous radiographs.

RESPIRATORY DISEASE AND OLDER PEOPLE

DEMOGRAPHICS

The population of many developed countries (European, North American and Australasian) is becoming elderly (Fig. 1). The management of these people in their 70s, 80s and older is increasingly routine. Unfortunately, few population studies have looked at respiratory disease in the elderly and even fewer have been pharmacological.

ASTHMA

Up to 10% of over 60-year-olds have wheezy breathlessness of asthma. However, most will have developed it before their 50s, and there is the possibility of several decades of well-managed through to unrecognised asthma. Hence, irreversible airway changes may have occurred.

Half of the deaths recorded for asthma are in the over 65-year-olds. This is partly explained by this age group forming such a large part of the population, but there is also a real and rising risk of death (UK Office of Population Census and Statistics). There has always been a risk of coding error with asthma and COPD deaths misaligned, though this source of error is now considered small.

COPD

As the lung ages, elastin tissue becomes less elastic. The age-related decline in lung function continues but alone is never enough to cause disability. The large numbers of individuals with COPD reflect previous smoking habits and occupational exposures. This is now the second commonest non-communicable chronic disease world-wide. Mortality as well as incidence is rising (Table 1), unlike the mortality due to stroke and coronary heart disease which is falling.

THERAPY

Few drug studies include the elderly or very elderly, and sometimes these individuals are positively excluded. To assume that drug effects are identical to younger individuals is trite. The

Table 1 **Trends in hospital admission rates for England and Wales for individuals aged 65 years and older for the two years 1994 and 2000.**

Disease	Rate/million 1994	2000	% change
COPD	5800	9700	+ 67
Pneumonia	4500	6000	+ 33
Interstitial lung diseases	120	250	+ 108

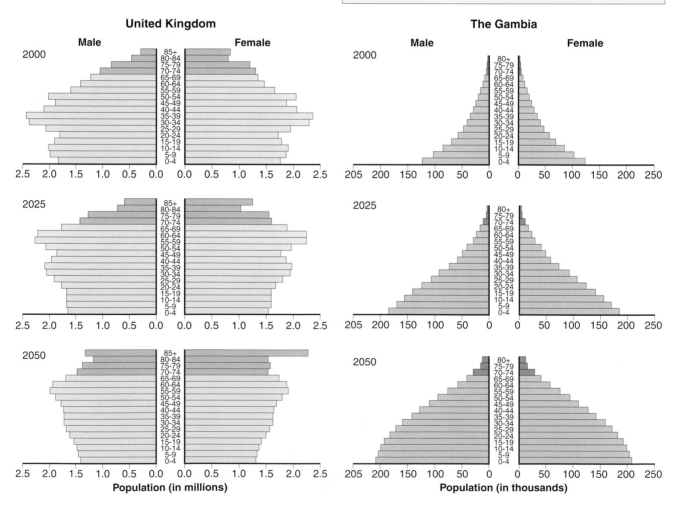

Fig. 1 **Population pyramids for the United Kingdom, The Gambia and China for 2000, and projected for 2025 and 2050.** These illustrate the population trends of developed and developing countries. A substantial population of individuals, mainly women over the age of 70 can be seen. (Source U.S. Census Bureau, International Data Base.)

Table 2 **Respiratory challenges in the elderly and common pitfalls**

Diagnosis:	increasing breathlessness attributed to increasing age alone or (simplistically) to bronchitis or heart failure.
Investigation:	should be appropriate.
Therapy:	co-morbidity more common with additional drug therapies. Hence, drug interactions and disease exacerbations more likely, for example non-steroidal anti-inflammatory drugs and ß-blocker eye drops exacerbating asthma. Finger arthritis will affect choice of inhaler device.
Prognosis:	longevity variable. Life expectancy at aged 71 for a male in the UK is 13 years, a decade later at age 81 it remains substantial at 7 years.

elderly patient may have a different lean body mass, different diet and dietary habits and ageing enzyme systems. Moreover, co-morbidities may result in other drug therapies with the potential for interaction. Impaired cognition may make therapy regimes inconsistently adhered too. If external agencies are involved in assisting therapy then the simplest effective regime will be required. Diminished dexterity including by arthritis will make the effective use of the ubiquitous metered-dose inhaler (MDI) impossible.

RESPIRATORY INFECTIONS

With a large prevalence of COPD, acute exacerbations including infections are frequent. Winter peaks of incidence and deaths tend to reflect respiratory viruses, including influenza, that are circulating in the communities.

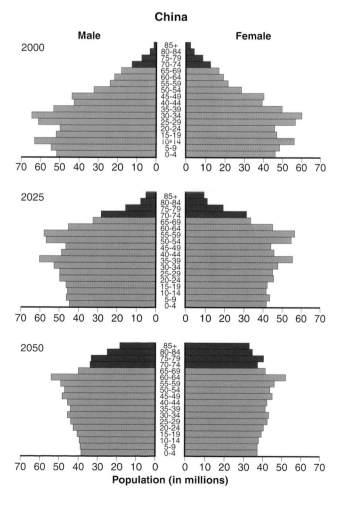

LUNG CANCER

A young person dying from lung cancer makes news. There is some evidence of a rising incidence in younger women of small cell lung cancer. Nevertheless, the majority of patients with lung cancer are elderly males suffering non-small cell lung cancer: a legacy of previous smoking habits and tobacco burning qualities. Occupational factors also contribute (Fig. 2).

Though there may be a tendency not to consider surgical resection or combination chemotherapy for the elderly, this is not based on evidence. With increasing age, performance status remains an important prognostic determinant but age does not. Lobectomy in the fit over-80s should be considered and also combination chemotherapy regimes in the over 75s. There is a hesitancy to use potent chemotherapy regimes because of a perception of reduced bone marrow reserves.

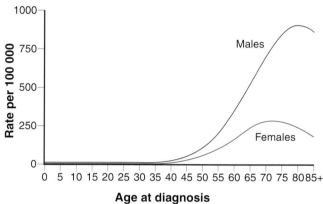

Fig. 2 **Age-specific rates for lung cancer in Scotland for the decade to 1995.** That it remains a disease predominantly of the elderly can be seen. (Reproduced from Harris V, Sandridge AL, Black RJ, Brewster DH, Gould A. Cancer Registration Statistics Scotland 1986–1995. Edinburgh: ISD Scotland Publications, 1998.)

Case history 34

An 85-year-old smoker is referred with deteriorating health and a spiculated mass apically situated on her chest radiograph. She had been told this was lung cancer but requested a second opinion. What would be appropriate?

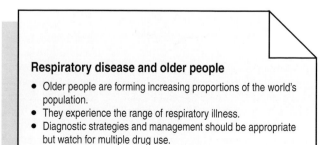

Respiratory disease and older people

- Older people are forming increasing proportions of the world's population.
- They experience the range of respiratory illness.
- Diagnostic strategies and management should be appropriate but watch for multiple drug use.

RESPIRATORY SERVICES

The effective and holistic care of patients with respiratory conditions, especially chronic, is improved by a team approach. Members of such a team may include:

RESPIRATORY NURSE SPECIALISTS

Nurses with additional specialist skills and knowledge can play a crucial part in the provision of quality care in both community and hospital respiratory practice. There are nationally approved courses of study and vocational qualifications are available in many specialist areas.

Asthma

Nurses with specialist training in asthma are the archetypal professional respiratory nurse. Their skills and experience allow them to undertake the tasks of communicating knowledge to patients, family members and healthcare colleagues and supporting the empowerment of patients. They should train and supervise patients' technique with delivery devices. Within appropriate protocols and clear responsibilities, giving advice on drug dose changes and even new drug prescribing are possible. These tasks are required as much in the community as in hospital.

Increasingly the benefits of nurse-supported and nurse-provided clinical services are clear to both healthcare professionals and patients alike.

Chronic obstructive pulmonary disease

The tasks for COPD may be similar to those performed for patients with asthma but additionally may include supervising domiciliary nebulisers and oxygen concentrators. Outreach ventures may include providing community support with drug therapy and loaned equipment for patients experiencing an exacerbation, thus providing welcome support as a 'hospital at home' or permitting an earlier supported discharge. Within a hospital-based service, nurses may have a central role in the initiation and supervision of non-invasive respiratory support.

Lung cancer

Supporting a patient and carers through the crucial time of diagnosis and breaking of bad news to at least commencement of any primary treatment are the chief responsibilities here. Other tasks may be the administration of chemotherapy, education of other healthcare workers and linking into a multidisciplinary team including community and palliative care professionals.

Tuberculosis contact tracing

This is performed by either full time nurses or identified and suitably trained health visitors. Following notification of a case of tuberculosis in the UK, a nurse will visit the index patient's address to discuss with them the following:

• their residence
• other individuals at the same address
• close contact colleagues in the workplace
• any regular visitors.

This information is reviewed for subsequent tracing and screening of contacts. Nurses should supervise treatment compliance, to the extent of directly observing drug consumption; in addition they should monitor clinic attendance and chase up defaulters.

Respiratory sleep disorders

Nurses are establishing new roles in this developing area. These include support and education of individuals with obstructive sleep apnoea, increasing involvement in troubleshooting interface problems and preparing patients for domiciliary-limited sleep studies.

RESPIRATORY PHYSIOTHERAPISTS

Primarily based in hospital providing an acute chest physiotherapy service, respiratory physiotherapists enjoy a wide variety of respiratory-related challenges.

Long-term supervision of patients with bronchiectasis, especially cystic fibrosis, may involve much community- and hospital-based work. Progressive exercise training programmes for patients with COPD and other chronic respiratory conditions develop cardio-pulmonary fitness, thereby maximising patients' physical abilities. This approach comes under the umbrella term of pulmonary rehabilitation.

Patients with the hyperventilation syndrome require an extended period of breathing re-training and relaxation exercises. Moreover, many patients with chronic asthma, COPD or other chronic respiratory diseases, including lung cancer, benefit from breathing relaxation training to help combat the distress and anxiety of breathlessness. Unless there is a large population base, this task may be performed by a trained physiotherapist in addition to other services.

RESPIRATORY PHYSIOLOGY MEASUREMENT TECHNICIANS

Maintenance of the equipment is crucial for reliable and meaningful results and also equipment survival. Their responsibilities may also include nebuliser or CPAP machine maintenance and patient training, teaching the correct use of delivery devices and participation in both undergraduate and postgraduate education programmes.

Direct access to spirometry measurements for patients of primary care physicians or the training of such physicians in the use of spirometers is an expanding opportunity. This particularly follows the importance of spirometry as stressed in recent guidelines for the diagnosis of COPD.

CHEST CLINIC

Here nurses, clerks, secretaries and radiographers provide a seamless support structure to allow physicians to assess and treat respiratory patients. This system evolved from a dedicated tuberculosis service and represents one of the first multidisciplinary, outpatient settings.

SMOKING CESSATION SUPPORT

Nurses, health educationalists and clinical psychologists provide counselling, support and pharmacological nicotine replacement therapy to individuals who wish to quit smoking.

OTHER HEALTHCARE PROFESSIONALS

Other healthcare professionals not already covered elsewhere include:
• Medical
— pulmonary oncologists
— palliative care physicians
• Professionals allied to medicine
— pharmacists
— occupational therapists
— dieticians
— social workers.

Respiratory services

• Modern medicine allows, and many patients and their carers demand, an holistic approach to a patient's respiratory condition.
• Team-playing is an important personal skill to acquire and develop.

SOURCES OF SUPPORT

This list is by no means exhaustive and is certainly more UK-specific. The commentary is purely my own.

ORGANISATIONS

British Thoracic Society (BTS)
17 Doughty Street
London
WC1N 2PL

Professional society welcoming nurses, physiotherapists and technicians. Source of professional standards, national guidance and national political promotion of respiratory medicine.

British Lung Foundation (BLF)
78 Hatton Garden
London EC1N 8JR

Fundraising charity which supports wide ranging respiratory research, supports patients and carers in regional 'Breathe Easy' clubs and generally promotes respiratory medicine

National Asthma Campaign (NAC)
Providence House
Providence Place,
London N1 0NT

Patient support and professional voice for asthma sufferers, carers and healthcare workers.

Roy Castle Lung Cancer Foundation
200 London Road
Liverpool L3 9TA

Specifically a lung cancer charity with fundraising and supported research, the latter around an International Lung Cancer Centre. Embraces mesothelioma too.

WEB SOURCES OF USEFUL INFORMATION

These web sites have been found informative and entertaining. They are aimed at a range of audiences including patients. Like so much on the web, these sites may change in quality, disappear or others may start with equal usefulness. I take no responsibility for such!

General organisations
www.lunguk.org
The BLF web site.

www.brit-thoracic.org uk
The BTS site.

www.ersnet.org
The European Respiratory Society site with e-journal and lectures that can be listened to complete with slides.

www.thoracic.org
Home page of the American Thoracic Society. Information and web links appropriate to both patients and professionals. Web-based learning resource too.

www.lungusa.org
American Lung Association, the lung health action group. Much useful information, patient support and links. Tobacco action and tuberculosis currently considered.

www.chss.org.uk
Chest Heart and Stroke Scotland, that provides information, support and small grants to help carers and patients with lung disease. Good little factsheets.

www.who.int/home-page
Home page for the World Health Organization that has information and reports often in relation to tuberculosis or other infectious diseases in developing countries.

www.cdc.gov
United States perspective that includes infectious diseases including tuberculosis and cancer registry information. Spotlights topical issues, US data and has links to related web sites. Includes self study modules including on tuberculosis.

www.phls.co.uk
Advice and facts on infectious diseases. Commendably not just an England and Wales perspective.

Cancer
www.roycastle.org
Roy Castle Foundation site.

www.cancerbacup.org.uk
Cancer site with a range of guidance on cancers, treatment and topical news. Not specific to lung cancer.

www.oncolink.com
Broad cancer information.

www.graylab.ac.uk/cancernet
Home page of Cancernet UK information database, a resource supported by the National Cancer Institute and BT. Valuable both to professionals and patients.

www.graylab.ac.uk/cancernet/ 201071.html
This is the address of the mesothelioma page in the Cancernet mentioned above. Lung cancer has many sites covering types and oncolytic therapies.

www.mesotheliomaweb.org
Specific mesothelioma information of interest to both professionals and patients.

www.imig.org
International mesothelioma interest group site.

Specific charities and action groups
www.asthma.org.uk
The NAC site.

www.cftrust.org.uk
Cystic fibrosis trust site limited to cystic fibrosis information, research, news and fundraising.

www.stoptb.org/home.html
Tuberculosis action group.

www.tbalert.org
Charity raising the profile of the action against tuberculosis. Good links page.

www.hht.org
HHT (Hereditary haemorrhagic telangiectasia) Foundation International website with support, education and information exchange.

http://lam.uc.edu
The LAM (lymphangioleiomyomatosis) homepage.

www.oeda.demon.co.uk
Covers asbestos and occupational issues. Pithy.

General information
www.sghms.ac.uk/depts/laia/laia.htm
Lung & Asthma Information Agency at St George's Hospital Medical School, London. Produces factsheets of contemporary data on a range of respiratory issues.

www.med.upenn.edu
Their 'hot topics' have some respiratory subjects with good images.

www.lumen.luc.edu/lumen/gme.htm
Graduate orientated but many respiratory topics covered in a pithy fashion.

www.priory.com/chest.htm
Chest medicine on-line. Submitted articles in a chatty style covering topical respiratory subjects from an English perspective.

RESPIRATORY TESTS AND TIPS

BRONCHIECTASIS: THE SACCHARIN TEST

Detection of either dysmotile cilia or abnormal mucus is by the saccharin test. Ensure that the individual is genetically able to taste saccharin.

A tiny fragment is then placed under direct vision upon one inferior turbinate (Fig. 1). The time taken for the individual to then taste the sweetness is recorded as a result of the saccharin molecules being carried into the naso-pharynx.

A normal individual will be able to taste the intense sweetness within 30 minutes.

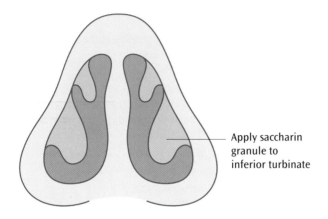

Apply saccharin granule to inferior turbinate

Fig. 1 **View up nostrils identifying site to place saccharin granule.**

ANTI-NEUTROPHIL CYTOPLASMIC ANTIBODIES

These are IgG auto-antibodies directed against one of two constituents or neutrophil cytoplasm: either myeloperoxidase (termed p-ANCA from artefactual perinuclear staining on cell preparations) or protease-3 (cytoplasmic staining, c-ANCA) (Fig. 2). ANCAs have been recognised as a characteristic serum autoantibody detectable in nearly 90% of patients with active Wegner's granulomatosis, especially c-ANCA which in high titre is closely associated with WG. Low levels of c-ANCA or the presence of p-ANCA is less specific, being present in other vasculitides and even non-vasculitic diseases.

Location of antibody binding		Likely antigen	Significance
c-ANCA	Cytoplasmic	Proteinase 3 (in granules)	• Present in high titre in majority of patients with Wegener's granulomatosis (80-90%) • Suppressed with adequate therapy, and may rise before clinical evidence of disease relapse • Pathogenic for Wegener's • Low levels may be present in many other vasculitides
p-ANCA	Perinuclear	Myeloperidoxidase (in granules)	• Variably present in many vasculitides and similar conditions, including Wegener's • For example SLE, Churg–Strauss • Significance in terms of diagnostic and therapeutic utility or pathogenesis unclear

Fig. 2 **Anti-neutrophil cytoplasmic antibodies and their significance.**

SKIN ALLERGY TESTING

Liquid extract introduced without awareness into skin. Label the sites on the skin (Fig. 3).

Use a range of relevant extracts and include positive (histamine) and negative controls. These may include house dust mite, cat, moulds, pollens, latex. Positive responses occur within 15 minutes with red, raised weals. Quantify response by measuring size of raised area.

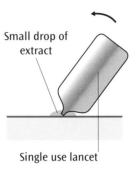

Small drop of extract

Single use lancet

Forearm marked, positive reactions visible

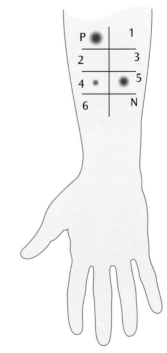

Fig. 3 **Skin allergy testing.** The lancet is rolled through the drop, pricking the skin.

ARTERIAL PUNCTURE FOR BLOOD GASES

Extend patient's elbow on support. Palpate the brachial artery and, aseptically, infiltrate a little volume of anaesthetic into the subcutaneous tissues ($\frac{1}{2}$ml of 1% lignocaine) (Fig. 4). Allow to work.

Puncture the artery by a direct perpendicular approach with a finebore needle. Deadspace of needle only filled with liquid heparin as an anticoagulant or use a pellet of dried heparin. Aim for a sample volume of more than 2ml.

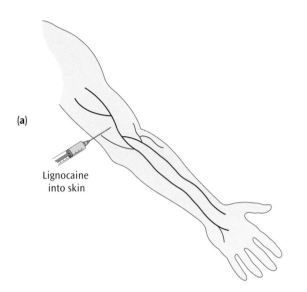

(a)

Lignocaine
into skin

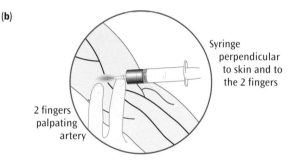

(b)

Syringe
perpendicular
to skin and to
the 2 fingers

2 fingers
palpating
artery

Fig. 4 **Arterial puncture for blood gas analysis.**

PEAK FLOW TESTING

Standing, full breath in, lips tight around the mouth piece and then blow out with a short sharp expiration, 'as if blowing out a candle' (Fig. 5). Beware of coughing that artificially increases the reading. Best of three readings made sequentially.

SPIROMETRY

Standing, full breath in, lips tight around mouth piece and then blow out as hard and as fast as possible, *but keep blowing* (Fig. 6). Repeat three times at least to yield similar traces. When FEV and FVC results suggest airflow limitation, it is worth repeating with three exhalations performed slowly, *relaxed* vital capacity.

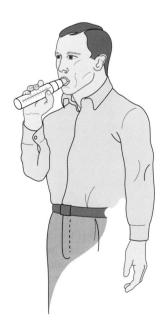

Fig. 5 **Measurement of peak expiratory flow rate.**

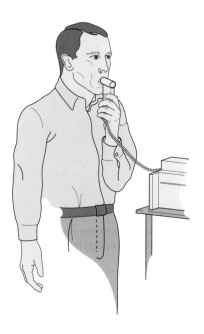

Fig. 6 **Spirometry, using an electronic flow meter and subsequent determination of volume to time.**

CASE HISTORY COMMENTS

Case history 1

Part of the nerve supply to the left vocal cord is the left recurrent laryngeal nerve. This travels down the side of the neck into the thorax to the level of the aortic arch before curving up to the larynx. In passing close to the lung hilum, it is susceptible to malignant compression or infiltration. The right cord is then moving against an immobile and unstressed left cord. This results in a weak 'bovine' cough and a change in voice quality.

Case history 2

This describes one of a minority of patients with substantial emphysema but with minimal airflow limitation. Perhaps tests of small airways, such as flow at mid-expiration, would have been impaired. The loss of parenchyma produces large spaces where gas diffusion to the alveolar–capillary membrane is the limiting factor. Thus, inadequate matching of gas delivery to perfusion explains the progressive hypoxia; initially apparent on exercise when the respiratory system is more challenged and then progressively impacts on resting gas exchange.

Case history 3

Acute hypoxia to the degree of peripheral cyanosis and such pulse oximetry readings would impair neurological function substantially, which it clearly has not. He is unlikely to have unrecognised chronic hypoxic lung disease or a congenital cyanotic heart deformation. Certain drugs cause reduction of circulating haemoglobin to methaemoglobin that has a blue appearance and typically produces false transcutaneous pulse oximetry readings of around 85%. Such drugs include dapsone.

Case history 4

The features in the history of a patient with asthma that you would wish to elicit include variable wheezy breathlessness, variability with well-known precipitants that include inhaled irritants. Though the nocturnal worsening would be in keeping with asthma, the lack of effect of other common precipitants and without even a partial relief to conventional therapy weighs against asthma. The most crucial feature of her story is the positional wheeze. Examination demonstrated an end-expiratory wheeze audible at her mouth and upper sternum, rather than the polyphonic wheeze to be expected in asthma. Subsequent bronchoscopy demonstrates a mobile polypoidal tracheal tumour attached via a narrow stalk.

Case history 5

With exertional breathlessness and cardiac murmurs, the cause of his breathlessness is most likely to be a heart valve. The findings are of aortic valve disease. Aortic regurgitation (the source of the immediate diastolic murmur) in particular tends to present late as a failing left ventricle and increasing pulmonary vascular congestion causes breathlessness and cough. This gentleman proceeded to valve replacement urgently.

Case history 6

With normal resting lung function, his severe breathlessness is not purely respiratory in origin. The interesting feature is that when on a bicycle (weight taken off his legs) he performed a large amount of work that he could not sustain when walking on a treadmill.

Indeed, the good exercise test performed on the bicycle suggests that he has good cardiopulmonary function. Perhaps his legs can not take the strain. Is he overweight? There is likely to be an emotional element too with the pending legal action. He weighed in at 105 kg at height 1.62 m.

Case history 7

This illustrates the importance of an adequate history and critical review of the available radiographic evidence in the light of that history (and any physical findings). Thoracic trauma was not mentioned on the radiograph request. The fractured rib seemingly was not conveyed to the GP, who requested a respiratory consult because of a pleural effusion.

Case history 8

Hoarseness and noisy breathing (stridor?) suggests laryngeal disease. Acute epiglottitis has to be the concern here. Though vaccination programmes have substantially reduced its incidence, non-immune adults and children can still present sporadically to practitioners. This lady rapidly progressed to airway obstruction that required urgent but difficult intervention by a skilled anaesthetist.

Case history 9

This is an apparent treatment failure in a severe pneumonia. The antibiotics are appropriate for the likely sensitivities of the known pathogen, but is methicillin-resistant *Staphylococcus* (MRSA) a possibility or are there others? Is there a complicating pleural empyema with the fever and pleurisy, or particularly with *Staphylococcus* or metastatic abscess formation? This lady was developing an empyema (also a septic shoulder arthritis)!

Case history 10

The Heaf skin test response following BCG vaccination would at most be expected to be a grade 2. A grade 4 response suggests other, and likely recent, mycobacterial infection even if no clinical disease is apparent.

Case history 11

This would be a Ports Authority and Public Health nightmare. Clearly, the immigrant needs counselling and commencement of supervised therapy at their place of residence and the case notified. Close co-passengers will need to be identified from the aircraft's passenger manifest, traced and counselled for screening. Staff should already be suitably protected and that recorded through their occupational medical support. Provision for the worried well should also be taken, perhaps a general notification to Public Health departments.

Case history 12

Highly significant. Risk factors for invasive pulmonary *Aspergillus* infection includes diabetes mellitus and intercurrent viral infection. The presence of staphylococcal infection makes one think of the latter. Indeed, influenza A antigen was identified in the bronchial washings with subsequently a rise in serological titre.

Case history 13

A diagnostic aspiration is required. I would suggest using a larger bore needle aseptically with a little local anaesthesia, anticipating pus.

Case history 14

The usual thought here with recurrent bronchitis would be asthma with perennial rhinitis. Airway obstruction is likely. However, on listening to her chest, the presence of predominately crackles rather than wheezes should prompt consideration of bronchiectasis. Thereafter at least think of a multi-system disorder. If she is Caucasian, a history of diabetes, gastrointestinal troubles or infertility should prompt a thought of cystic fibrosis. Ciliary dysfunction may be more likely if there is just respiratory tract involvement with infertility difficulties.

Case history 15

Obtain some sputum, using hypertonic nebulised saline as he does not have a productive cough. A peripheral blood count with a differential white cell count and a mouth examination looking for oral thrush would be prudent. Though he may be immuno-competent or have a conventional pneumonia, *Pneumocystis carinii* pneumonia may present this way.

Case history 16

His smoking may well have caused airways obstruction as COPD. However many joiners, particularly those who have worked in industrial premises, will have had exposure to asbestos. Whether this has been heavy enough to cause asbestosis suggested by lung fibrosis as basal crackles, will have to be determined by asking him. Any such exposure may also have contributed to airway disease.

Case history 17

Immediate thoughts are of farmer's lung, an extrinsic allergic alveolitis caused by exposure to fungi in haylofts. However, it is always important to revise exposures with the patient. This individual owned a large arable farm, kept a few Highland cattle for showing but had also dabbled in pigeon breeding over the preceding 18 months. It was the birds!

Case history 18

The radiographs and high resolution CT suggest sarcoidosis. However, widespread lung crackles would be uncommon in sarcoidosis, even with widespread chest radiographic abnormalities. The issues of weight loss and cardiopulmonary fitness as contributors to his breathlessness require addressing too, particularly as he may require treatment with corticosteroids.

Case history 19

A number of diagnostic possibilities present themselves. These range from the non-vasculitides of intercurrent infection with over-anticoagulation to a vasculitis with lung haemorrhage and renal involvement. Urine for microscopy with blood for immunology, autoantibodies including ANCAs and eosinophil count are required as a minimum. Consider reversing the anticoagulation, and mechanical respiratory support may be required.

Case history 20

Clearly yes, this is a common style of presentation. The night disturbance is typical and no wonder he is tired during the day: underachieving at school. Is he unfit or, more likely, has he a degree of exercise-induced asthma? He should be able to measure his peak flow rates: morning and evening with extra readings at times of symptoms. If this does not show the expected variability, then an exercise challenge with readings before and frequently after a period of running.

Case history 21

A number of precipitants must be considered. Has he started to smoke or has he moved accommodation, perhaps sharing with a smoker? Has he acquired a pet? Has he started a new job and is developing an occupational component? Is he still using his treatment?

Case history 22

He clearly has airways obstruction on current spirometry. The history of breathlessness suggests chronicity, though any previous spirometry recordings would be valuable. With a smoking history of 50 pack-years this is sufficient to suggest a diagnosis of chronic obstructive pulmonary disease. Any childhood symptoms or those of atopy that would suggest reversible airways disease of asthma, when reversibility should be looked for and treated aggressively. Eighteen months later a chest radiograph was required, as a complicating malignancy was the concern.

Case history 23

He has airways obstruction with gas trapping clinical and radiological. A trivial smoker, if this was COPD you must consider a_1-anti-trypsin deficiency. The clue here is his occupation. Firemen may be exposed to a range of noxious chemicals, including products of combustion. Nitric oxides of nitrogen are commonly produced when plastics burn (with volatile cyanides). They can cause airways obstruction as an obliterative bronchiolitis.

Case history 24

This case is an example of lung cancer presenting with symptoms other than respiratory. The most useful tests are likely to be bronchoscopy and biopsy. However, a PA and lateral chest radiograph at least must be reviewed to be sure that the mass is central and hence likely to be accessed by bronchoscopy. It may just be subpleural when a percutaneous approach for biopsy would then be best.

The pain is of recent duration and there is no mention of trauma. Thus the concern is that he has a metastasis from the lung cancer in his hip or left pelvis. A plain radiograph of the area may show bone loss, as a 'lytic' lesion is likely. An isotope bone scan is almost certain to demonstrate increased isotope uptake, a 'hot' spot. Demonstration of metastatic cancer may at times obviate the need to pursue confirmation of the primary site.

The low serum sodium suggests the presence of small cell lung cancer with inappropriate ADH secretion. Importantly his serum calcium is normal. This must be checked in individuals with malignancy and bone pain or confusion (? hypercalcaemia). The elevated alkaline phosphatase is in keeping with the bone metastasis and reflects the osteoblastic activity at that bone site. It may just reflect liver metastases too.

Case history 25

Metastatic bone pain is well relieved by a mix of anti-inflammatory non-steroidal analgesic and strong opiate analgesia.

Bisphosphonates may have a place in recalcitrant pain. External beam irradiation should be arranged.

Case history 26

Further investigation for confirmation is required, before embarking on longer-term anticoagulation that is not without risk. Either an isotope perfusion lung scan or CT pulmonary angiography is required, depending on local resources. If either is non-contributory to the diagnosis then indirect evidence should be sought. The diagnostic utility of an elevated plasma D-dimer assay is of increasing interest. Leg vein imaging for deep leg vein thrombosis or right heart echocardiography for pulmonary hypertension would be the next steps. If pulmonary embolisation is confirmed the contraceptive pill is contraindicated. She should cease it and use alternative means of contraception.

Case history 27

The rapid development of a substantial shunt in this setting is typically due to pulmonary fat emboli. It is too soon for the development of venous thrombosis and subsequent embolisation. In view of the thoracic trauma, a pneumothorax must be considered and actively sought too.

Case history 28

It is likely the trauma cracked a rib and caused a pneumothorax. The pleural air would have expanded in volume as the ambient pressure fell in the aircraft cabin as it gained altitude. This expansion would compromise further ventilation and cardiac output. There is a real risk of the pneumothorax tensioning. Though urgent intervention to decompress the pleural space is required, she should not have flown in the first instance.

Case history 29

This lady should undergo diagnostic pleural aspiration and biopsy. Aspiration of 1.5 litres of fluid will ease her breathlessness. Unless she is very frail, I would certainly discuss with her the merits of formal tube drainage and a talc or tetracycline pleurodesis to try to prevent fluid re-accumulation.

Case history 30

This man now requires an overnight sleep study with a reasonable clinical concern of obstructive sleep apnoea. The case touches upon the breadth of referral patterns as patients may present themselves to many different specialists including occupational physicians and neurologists.

Case history 31

Difficulty in weaning should always prompt the consideration as to whether the biochemical milieu of the muscles is adequate. The information provided demonstrates a low serum phosphate and low potassium. Both serum levels represent significant deficiencies of the ions that are necessary for adequate skeletal muscle function. Moreover, the difficulties noted in attempting to restore serum potassium should prompt a concern that he is magnesium deplete too. Typically, hypomagnesaemia is associated with hypokalaemia and will require correcting before restoration of potassium levels is possible. Trace elements and essential fatty acids may be depleted too. Chronic alcoholism is likely to be the reason: inadequate dietary intake and increased losses through alcohol-induced diuresis and alcohol-associated diarrhoea.

Case history 32

Lung volume reduction surgery is an alternative to lung transplantation, without the problem of lack of donors. Subjective benefit is derived without much change in readily measurable physiology, reflecting in part the relative insensitivity of such tests. The benefit is due to repositioning the respiratory muscle pump into a mechanically more advantageous position.

Case history 33

The clinical pattern of deterioration with drop in ambient pressure and recovery upon aircraft descent is in keeping with a fixed gas volume within the thorax. This would expand with a fall in ambient pressure and constrict as the ambient pressure rose (Boyle's gas law). Hence, this gentleman had suffered his (first) spontaneous pneumothorax. A chest radiograph confirmed a modest (at sea level) pneumothorax.

Case history 34

Review of the radiology demonstrated a single shadow situated subpleurally. She agreed to and underwent CT guided lung biopsy with material dispatched fresh for culture as well as in fixative for histology. Caseation was demonstrated and in due course mycobacterium malmoense was grown. She gradually recovered over the first 6 months of a 24-month course of anti-mycobacterial chemotherapy.

Note
All the above case histories are based on real clinical dilemmas.

INDEX